ROUTLEDGE LIBRARY E]
SCOTLAND

Volume 13

SURVIVAL OF THE UNFITTEST

SURVIVAL OF THE UNFITTEST
A Study of Geriatric Patients in Glasgow

BERNARD ISAACS, MAUREEN LIVINGSTONE
AND YVONNE NEVILLE

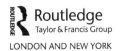

Routledge
Taylor & Francis Group

LONDON AND NEW YORK

First published in 1972 by Routledge & Kegan Paul

This edition first published in 2022
by Routledge
2 Park Square, Milton Park, Abingdon, Oxon OX14 4RN

and by Routledge
605 Third Avenue, New York, NY 10158

Routledge is an imprint of the Taylor & Francis Group, an informa business

British Library Cataloguing in Publication Data
A catalogue record for this book is available from the British Library

ISBN: 978-1-03-206184-9 (Set)
ISBN: 978-1-00-321338-3 (Set) (ebk)
ISBN: 978-1-03-207787-1 (Volume 13) (hbk)
ISBN: 978-1-03-207795-6 (Volume 13) (pbk)
ISBN: 978-1-00-321157-0 (Volume 13) (ebk)

DOI: 10.1201/9781003211570

Publisher's Note
The publisher has gone to great lengths to ensure the quality of this reprint but points out that some imperfections in the original copies may be apparent.

Disclaimer
The publisher has made every effort to trace copyright holders and would welcome correspondence from those they have been unable to trace.

Survival of the Unfittest

A study of geriatric patients in Glasgow

Bernard Isaacs
Maureen Livingstone
Yvonne Neville

Routledge & Kegan Paul
London and Boston

First published 1972
by Routledge and Kegan Paul Ltd
Broadway House,
68-74 Carter Lane,
London, EC4V 5EL and
9 Park Street, Boston, Mass. 02108, U.S.A.
Printed in Great Britain by
The Lavenham Press Ltd
ISBN 0 7100 7233 3

Contents

		page
Introduction		ix

Part I

1	The Fall of Mrs McGoldrick	1
2	The East End of Glasgow	4
3	The Evolution of the Geriatric Service	8
4	The Hard Core	16
5	The Co-ordinates of Care	23
6	Insufficient Basic Care	28
7	The Anatomy of Neglect: Preoccupation	34
8	The Anatomy of Neglect: Dilemma, Refusal	40
9	The Anatomy of Neglect: Rejection	45
10	The Bonds of Strain	50
11	The Sources of Strain	55
12	The Victims of Strain	63
13	The Triangles of Dependency	71

14   Incontinence   78

15   Community Care   84

16   'Something Must Be Done'   93

Part II
Materials and Methods; Definitions   104

Appendices   114

Tables   126

Bibliography   162

Index   167

Figures

		page
1	Concept of the 'hard core'	21
2	Reasons for acceptance to the geriatric unit	24
3	The spectrum of need	26
4	Factors influencing admission of geriatric patients	35
5	The triangles of dependency	76
6	Changes in the structure of the population of Scotland aged sixty-five and over from the Registrar General's reports and projection	77

Introduction

This book aims to tell the story of ill old people in the East End of Glasgow as we observed them during our researches in the late 1960s. Detailed accounts of our surveys have been published in scientific periodicals; but in this volume we have brought these studies together, expanded them, and drawn general conclusions from them about the plight of ill old people in a modern urban society. The social and economic circumstances of the East End of Glasgow differ widely from those prevailing in other parts of the United Kingdom, and in urban communities in other countries; but essentially this book is about people, and it seems very likely that in all societies people behave with the same compassion towards one another in times of suffering as we found amongst the elderly and their families in Glasgow. In the case histories which illustrate our narrative fictitious names and addresses have been used. Details of methods and results are set out separately in the second part of the book, but references to them are provided in the main text. It is hoped that the book will interest doctors, nurses, social workers, ancillary workers, administrators, politicians and voluntary workers who are involved in providing services for the elderly, and also those whose concern for the aged sick stems from their own experience of caring for an ill old person.

The surveys on which the book is based were supported by a grant from the Research and Intelligence Unit of the Scottish Home and Health Department. Dr M. A. Heasman, Director of the Unit, and Dr W. Thom of the Scottish Home and Health Department have taken an extremely close interest in the work from planning to completion, and the authors are deeply indebted to them for a wealth of advice and practical assistance.

In the field work of the surveys and the analysis of data the authors were most fortunate in having the services of the following people, whose major contribution to the study is warmly acknowledged: Dr William Matheson, Mrs Catherine Campbell, Mr John Browning, Miss Isobel McMillan, Mr Andrew McKechan, Mrs Alexandrina Lang and Mrs Joanne Abbott.

Throughout the surveys the patients and subjects, their relatives, their family doctors and receptionists collaborated in our enquiries with great kindness and frankness. Generous co-operation was also obtained from the superintendents and records officers of the Glasgow hospitals to whom a stream of queries were addressed. We also wish to record with great pleasure our thanks to the following who did a great deal to assist our studies: Dr C. Bainbridge, Senior Administrative Medical Officer, Western Regional Hospital Board; Mr A. A. MacIver, Secretary and Treasurer, Glasgow Royal Infirmary and Associated Hospitals; Dr A. R. Miller, Medical Officer of Health, City of Glasgow; Mr T. Tinto, lately Secretary and Principal Welfare Officer of the former Health and Welfare Department, City of Glasgow; Dr W. W. Fulton, Secretary, Glasgow Local Medical Committee; Mr T. H. Souter, Clerk, Executive Council, City of Glasgow; Dr S. Iversen, Medical Statistics Department, Western Regional Hospital Board; The Clerks of the Executive Councils of Dunbartonshire, Lanarkshire, Renfrewshire, Stirlingshire and other areas; The Consultant Physicians of Glasgow Royal Infirmary; The Registration Section of the former Health and Welfare Department, Corporation of Glasgow; The Librarians of the Mitchell Library, Commercial Library and of the Royal College of Physicians and Surgeons of Glasgow; and Mr G. Munday and Mr I. C. F. Oak, lately of the Scottish Hospitals' Computer Centre.

During the project a great deal of extra work fell on colleagues, and particular thanks are due to Dr Malcolm Fletcher and Mrs Myra Dykes. Thanks are also expressed to the editor of the *Scottish Medical Journal* for his permission to print Figures 1 and 2 which were first published in the *Scottish Medical Journal* (1969) vol. 14, p. 243 in the article, 'Some characteristics of geriatric patients' and to the editor of the *British Medical Journal* for his permission to print Figure 3 which was first published in the *British Medical Journal* (1971) vol. 4, p. 282 in the article, 'Geriatric patients: do their families care?'.

Part I

1 The Fall of Mrs McGoldrick

At 1.30 a.m. on 1 October 1966 Mrs Bridget McGoldrick aged eighty-six rose from bed in her home in Glasgow's East End to use the toilet, and fell. She struggled to rise to her feet, but she was too weak to do so, and soon became exhausted by her efforts. She did not try to shout for help because there was no one to hear her. She lived alone and did not wish to disturb the neighbours; in any case she realized that her feeble cries would not be heard through the thick stone walls. And so she lay all night long on the cold floor of the unheated room.

Her home was on the top storey of a four-floor tenement building. It consisted of a single room, barely furnished, and equipped with a box-bed built into a recess in the wall, and a sink with a cold water tap only. The toilet was situated on a landing halfway down the outside staircase, and was shared by the three households on the top floor of the building.

Mrs McGoldrick had lived here for more than sixty years. In this little house her eight children had been born and reared, and from here she had left to bury three of them who died in infancy or childhood. From here, too, her husband had gone out to his work, or to tramp the streets of Glasgow when no work was to be found. He had returned drunk and jubilant when, as she suspected, he had won at the horses or the dogs, or sullen and violent when his fortune turned. Then he too had died, while still a young man, and she had to go out cleaning offices to earn a few shillings, a job in which she had continued until the age of seventy-two, when she was forced by her 'rheumatics' to give it up. From the same home she had said goodbye to her children who had emigrated to Canada in search of a better life, or who had found jobs in England. Now only her youngest daughter was left, but she too had moved recently to the new town of Cumbernauld, where life for her four children was good, and work was to be had, but rents and bus fares into Glasgow were high.

Mrs McGoldrick had been confined to the house by osteoarthritis for nearly three years. The stairs were quite beyond her, and she had even had to give up using the outside lavatory. For toilet purposes she used a bucket kept under the bed, and she depended on her neighbours and her home help to empty this for her. Once, a long time ago, her doctor had wanted her to have an X-ray to see if anything could be done but she had refused, because, so she thought, 'What can anyone do for me at my age?' The doctor still came to see her every now and again and gave her pills which helped her, but gradually she found it more and more difficult to cope. Getting out of bed to use her bucket at night was the worst thing, but she could not understand how, on this occasion, she had missed her footing. But there she lay. The night was cold and windy and she was covered only by a thin nightdress. Her limbs ached, she was sick with the pain and shock of her fall, exhausted by her struggles and desperate to pass water. But she offered up a prayer and composed herself for the long lonely vigil.

At 9 a.m. on the morning of 1 October 1966 the home help came to the door and let herself in with her own key. She found Mrs McGoldrick icy cold, bruised and stiff, lying where she had fallen, but fully conscious. She ran to the neighbours for help, and together they lifted her into bed, gave her warm drinks and summoned the doctor.

At 10 a.m. the telephone rang in the office of the Department of Geriatric Medicine of Glasgow Royal Infirmary Group of Hospitals. It was Mrs McGoldrick's doctor seeking her urgent admission to hospital. The secretary replied, 'I am afraid we have no vacant beds and cannot take her in right away, but I shall ask the consultant to visit the house today, and we will do the best we can for her. If you think she cannot wait please try to have her admitted as an emergency to the Royal Infirmary.'

For the geriatric department this was a routine referral, typical of the many hundreds of requests received each year from general practitioners for the admission of elderly patients to hospital. But it was also a very special one. It was, by chance, the first case to be included in a systematic analysis of all patients referred to the geriatric unit during the fifteen-month period which started on 1 October 1966. The objects of this study were threefold: first, to analyse the patients who were referred to the department—their personal, family, domestic, social and medical circumstances, the measures taken to assist them, and the outcome of their treatment; second, to convey to others something of the anguish and misery endured by the aged sick and their relatives; and third, to seek better ways of dealing in the future with the problems which the study revealed.

The rest of Mrs McGoldrick's tale is quickly told. She was admitted, after a brief interval, to the geriatric unit; during the waiting period her daughter, the neighbours and the home help combined to give her the necessary attention. She was weak and confused and was found to have developed pneumonia, from which she slowly recovered after treatment. But she never regained even her former level of health, and although she was walking about the ward within a month of her admission, she was obviously unfit to return to her own home or to enter an Eventide Home. She refused to consider going to live with her daughter, whose house was in any case too small to accommodate her, and she was eventually transferred to a long-stay geriatric ward where she remained semi-ambulant, trying to give no one any trouble, until her death two years later.

It is with the report of this survey of patients referred to the geriatric unit that this book is mainly concerned; underlying it is the conviction that Mrs McGoldrick, lying on the floor of her house throughout the wintry night, symbolizes a social evil. How has this, and the many other cases of deprivation in the aged, been allowed to come about in the midst of a welfare state, and what can we do to ensure that such things do not continue to happen? The conclusions which emerged from the studies can be summarized here. What we are witnessing in the 'developed' societies of today is something that has never existed before on the present scale in human history: it is the Survival of the Unfittest. The advances made in this century by medicine and the social services have combined to reverse a biological law. No longer are the unfit eliminated; instead they are nurtured and protected. Man, alone among the animals, is now provided with the means of survival in a state of unfitness. It is now normal for life to close, as it began, with a period of prolonged dependency; but whereas we have for long organized our society to care for the helpless infant and the developing child, we are only beginning to seek means of dealing with the problems created by dependency in old age. Mrs McGoldrick lay helpless on the floor, not because her family neglected her, not because there was a shortage of hospital beds or residential homes, but because the full implication of the biological change that has been taking place in these last two or three decades has yet to be grasped.

2   The East End of Glasgow

The East End of Glasgow, where Mrs McGoldrick lived, fans out from its apex near the Royal Infirmary to its base beyond the city boundary. It can be divided into three areas, which might be called the Near East, the Middle East and the Far East.

The Near East is the Glasgow of the industrial revolution, when the massive housing needs of the population, swollen by influxes from the surrounding countryside, from the Highlands of Scotland and from Ireland, were met by the erection of street after street of grim tenements. These slums are giving way to new blocks of tall flats, but in 1967 many thousands of people still inhabited the crumbling tenements. The majority of these were buildings of four storeys with three households to each floor; but sometimes there were two, sometimes four. Most of these houses consisted of a single room or a 'room and kitchen', although in some of the better tenements larger houses were to be found. In the older tenements there were no baths, no running hot water supply and no inside toilets. The toilets were to be found in a little alcove halfway down the staircase, and each served the needs of the two, three or four households on the landing. The stairs were usually straight, but the oldest buildings had a turret built out at the back containing a spiral staircase on which the toilets were located. The families living on the ground floor had the toilets on the same level, but ground floor accommodation was unpopular with the elderly, who feared burglars and the depredations of children.

The houses were approached through the typical Scottish 'close', which is a doorless, stone-lined passage, open at the front to the street and at the back to the 'back court'—a muddy or stony courtyard behind the houses, where children played, clothes were dried and refuse was collected. The houses were damp and draughty and boasted few amenities. In those which had never been modernized the

4

characteristic features of the old Glasgow working-class house were still to be seen—the low zinc sink with its wooden draining board and brass swan-neck cold tap, the black grate with its open coal fire, perhaps one or two gas rings or the old gas cooker, and the high box-bed built into the bed recess. However, many houses had been at least partially modernized, with tiled fireplaces, gas or electric fires, modern gas or electric cookers and water heaters, while the bed recess had been turned into a dinette, and a low divan bed had been installed.

The ground floor of many of these blocks contained shops—a dairy, a general store, a newsagent's and confectioner's or a public house. They were close to main streets and public transport.

Not so long ago it was common for these houses to be occupied by a husband and wife and some six, eight or ten children, or even more. By 1967 most large families had moved away, fewer young people were left, and a large proportion of the tenement houses were occupied by old people living alone, or by elderly couples. Most of the men had been semi-skilled or unskilled labourers; some were skilled men who had descended in the social scale as a result of unemployment, ill health or alcohol. The old people grumbled about vandalism, damp and the price of coal, but they looked in on one another, kept each other company, met on the stairs and at the shops, performed little services for one another, or just looked out of the window on the life of the street below.

A little further east the tenement houses were larger, with two, three or four rooms, a toilet, and sometimes even a bathroom. The close was tiled; in the back court a few blades of grass sprouted. In some houses the toilets seemed to have been added as a novelty or an afterthought, for some were elevated on a little throne, others were located inside a cupboard or in an L-shaped space left over when the other rooms were completed. They posed hazards to the elderly users, almost as great as those of the outside staircase.

An island of middle-class housing, once a desirable residential suburb and still containing some fine villas and terrace houses, lay in the heart of the Near East, and provided the survey with a small number of patients in the Registrar General's social classes I and II.

The Middle East consisted mainly of a large Corporation housing estate built between the wars. The houses were of cottage type or four-in-a-block, with trim gardens and garages. The streets had grass verges and trees. Most of the tenants had occupied these houses for twenty-five or thirty years, and some had lived there since the houses were built forty years before. The old people now under-occupied their three or four-apartment houses. Most were skilled tradesmen and engineers, who built the Clyde's great ships and locomotives. They displayed framed photographs of their sons and daughters graduating from university, or playing with suntanned children on the beaches of Vancouver or Sydney.

The Far East was a huge area of post-war housing estates. The houses here were mostly designed for young two-generation families, and were of three or four apartments. Most of them were in three- or four-storey walk-up tenements, but there were also a few multi-storey blocks. In 1967 there were few shops in the area, no pubs, no cinemas or dance halls and few opportunities for social activity, despite the excellent work of the churches and voluntary organizations. Residents complained frequently about the transport services.

Specially designed pensioners' houses, mostly dating from the 1950s and grouped in little clusters of twelve or twenty, were scattered throughout the Middle and Far East. They had a kitchen, a bathroom, and a single large living-room-cum-bedroom, sometimes with a dividing screen. Some were grouped in much larger blocks of up to 100 houses, with a resident caretaker who did not, however, provide the services associated with purpose-built warden-service flatlets. The residents of these blocks sat outside together in the summer sunshine, or called on each other with plates of soup in the winter. They sat at their windows and watched the arrival of the mobile shop, the children running to the ice-cream van at the sound of the chiming bells, the ambulance calling for one of their number, or the hearse.

The population of the eight electoral wards which comprise the East End of Glasgow was about 248,000, according to the 10 per cent sample census of 1966 (Table 1, p. 126). This was about one-quarter of the population of the City of Glasgow. There were 22,600 people in the East End who were aged sixty-five or over. This was 9 per cent of the population, compared with 10 per cent for the City of Glasgow as a whole, 11 per cent for the whole of Scotland, and 12 per cent for England and Wales. In the individual electoral wards the percentage aged sixty-five and over ranged from 6 per cent in the post-war housing area to 15 per cent in the old tenement areas.

According to the 1966 census, in the East End of Glasgow there was a population density of thirty-seven persons to the acre. This compared with twenty-four for the City of Glasgow as a whole, nineteen for London and twenty-one for Birmingham. In the various wards of the East End the density ranged from eighteen persons per acre in the post-war housing schemes to fifty-six per acre in the oldest tenement area.

The eastern area of Glasgow in 1967 was a highly urbanized, densely populated, poorly housed area. The low proportion of old people in the population was due partly to the inclusion of the large post-war housing area occupied mainly by younger families, and partly to the high mortality in middle life of the generation who now constitute the elderly population and to their high migration rate. The old people have lived through two world wars and the intervening depression. Poor housing, atmospheric pollution, poverty and subnutrition took their toll of them, but those who survived lived their lives packed tightly together in the smoke and slums, and acquired a toughness, mutual respect and devotion which stood them in good stead in their later years.

3 The Evolution of the Geriatric Service

The pattern of the health services available to the populace of the eastern area of Glasgow in 1967 was that of the tripartite structure of the National Health Service. The family doctor provided first-line care; the Local Authority was responsible for preventive and domiciliary services; and the Regional Hospital Board controlled a number of general and specialized hospitals.

The family doctor provided his services free of charge. Patients could be seen in their own homes or at the doctors' surgeries with the minimum of formality. Yet many old people were reluctant to turn to their doctors for help. Perhaps they recalled the days before 1948 when the uninsured—a group which included the wife and family of the workers—had to pay the doctor one shilling for a consultation and one and sixpence for a visit. From this a tradition had grown up 'never to trouble the doctor unless you have to'.

Before the National Health Service, Glasgow, like other large cities, had a dual hospital system. On the one hand were the great voluntary hospitals, like Glasgow Royal Infirmary, with their long traditions, their large endowments, and their prestige as centres of teaching and research. They attracted well-educated nurses, and they taught medical students who competed keenly for the lowly-paid house-doctor posts. To obtain an honorary appointment in a voluntary hospital was the mark of professional attainment, and the key to material and social success. The captains of industry and the leading professional men of the city were proud to serve on the committees of management.

The hospitals belonging to the Public Health Department of the Corporation of Glasgow were somewhat less prestigious places. The Corporation had sole responsibility for the hospital treatment of infectious diseases and tuberculosis, and they also operated two large and two small general hospitals. In the educational qualifications of their nurses, in their level of medical staffing, and in their social status the Corporation hospitals were inferior to the voluntary hospitals. Indeed, it was a not unusual practice for a physician holding a relatively junior appointment in a voluntary hospital to be in charge of wards in a Corporation hospital.

The first major change in status of the Corporation hospitals took place in 1936 with the establishment in Stobhill Hospital, jointly by the Public Health Department of Glasgow Corporation and the University of Glasgow, of the clinical teaching unit of the Regius Professor of Materia Medica and Therapeutics.

The two types of hospital differed in their selection of patients and in the administrative arrangements for their admission. The voluntary hospitals exercised the right to choose. They were always ready to admit the young and the acutely ill, but were reluctant to accept too many chronic sick and elderly patients lest their function as centres of teaching and research be jeopardized. The Corporation hospitals exercised no selection. Their beds were open to all who came, and the elderly, the socially downcast and the chronically ill formed a high proportion of their patients.

This polarization of 'acute' cases into voluntary hospitals and 'chronic' into municipal hospitals was aided by the different admission arrangements. If a general practitioner wanted to have a patient admitted to a voluntary hospital he had to telephone the receiving house physician and justify the patient's admission on the grounds not only that he was ill but also that he was 'suitable'. The criteria of suitability were presumably conveyed to the house physician by his chief, and there was something of a suspicion that in some wards at least they reflected the research and teaching interests of the staff as much as the needs of the patient. A question always asked was, 'How old is the patient?', and some general practitioners of considerable standing were made to feel, by a freshly qualified house physician, that they had committed a social misdemeanour in applying for the admission of a patient over the age of sixty.

With the Corporation hospitals it was all much easier. Admissions were arranged through the Hospital Admissions Department, known universally as the 'Bar'. The Bar was the reception desk of the Public Health Department. This name appears to have been given to the broad counter separating the public without from the clerks within by the first sanitary inspectors who worked in the building. They were retired policemen and carried the terminology of their former profession with them. A doctor wishing to have a patient admitted to a Corporation hospital simply gave the name, age and diagnosis to the clerk at the Bar, and left him to get on with the job. There were no difficulties, no delays, no embarrassing questions, and no need even to order the ambulance. Some doctors merely scribbled a note, handed it to the relatives and said, 'Here, take this down to the Bar'.

The voluntary hospitals took some cases from the Bar, but this was not a commitment, and when things were busy the house physician 'closed the ward to the Bar'. The placement of patients referred to the Bar, although it was largely conducted by clerks, was supervised by doctors assisted by visiting nurses. But the general effect of this dual admission system was that the tradition grew up among the medical profession that 'acute' cases were sent into voluntary hospitals, while municipal hospitals were for the chronic sick. Doctors holding appointments simultaneously in the two types of hospital acquired the habit of transferring patients who required long-term hospital care from their beds in the voluntary hospital to their municipal hospital wards.

Another feature of the hospital scene in the city was Barnhill, a huge grim Poor Law Institution with a large ill-equipped hospital section. This building passed into the administration of the Corporation in 1929. Cases were admitted to the hospital section of Barnhill from the residential accommodation there, known as the 'Body of the House', and also by transfer from other hospitals, mainly those run by the Corporation. There was little or no active medical treatment in the modern sense, and Barnhill was looked upon by the general hospitals as a suitable place for the terminal care of the irremediable, or, not to put too fine a point on it, as a 'dumping-ground'.

Psychiatric services were provided by a ring of immense Victorian mental hospitals in isolated positions on the periphery of the city. The admission of old people to these wards was arranged by the duly authorized officer of the Local Authority on the application of the general practitioner or the family, and usually on the basis of socially unacceptable behaviour with no precise medical diagnosis. Of active treatment there was, in those days, little, and elderly patients admitted to mental hospitals generally remained there until they died.

Three of the Corporation general hospitals had mental observation wards in which non-certified psychiatric cases were investigated and treated, and were then either discharged or were transferred to the mental hospitals.

In theory, the National Health Service put all the city general hospitals on the same footing. All were now expected to admit any ill person in their area. The ex-Corporation hospitals developed out-patient clinics, increased their staff, improved their training of nurses, involved themselves in undergraduate and postgraduate medical education, and struggled to acquire the prestige of 'acute hospitals'. Meantime, many changes were taking place in the face of medicine. 'Acute medicine' was becoming increasingly scientific and specialized. New skills and techniques were being developed. The voluntary hospitals were anxious to retain their position in the forefront of medical advance, and the ex-Corporation hospitals were keen not to lag behind. New units sprang up for cardiological surgery, acute coronary care, renal dialysis, intensive care and many other specialties. The needs of these services created intense pressure in acute medical units, and elderly and chronic sick patients were seen as a threat to the efficient running of acute wards. Increasingly the ex-Corporation hospitals drew their patients from their own new outpatient clinics, and from direct contact with general practitioners in the area. The function of the Bar changed, until it dealt almost entirely with the elderly and the chronic sick. And all this time the number of old people in the population was rising.

The situation in Glasgow was similar to that which obtained throughout the country. Already in 1948 the word 'geriatrics' was being heard in Glasgow. Pioneering work in the field was being undertaken by the late Dr Marjorie Warren, Lord Amulree, Dr Thomas Wilson and others; Professor Noah Morris, the first occupant of the university unit at Stobhill Hospital, had been an early and powerful advocate of the establishment of acute geriatric units for the precise diagnosis and treatment of disease in old age.

In 1949 the first geriatric unit in Glasgow was set up at the Southern General Hospital, an ex-Corporation hospital under Dr O. T. Brown. This was a highly successful experiment in using modern methods of medical care for the aged and the chronic sick, but the unit was small, with few resources, and was able to do little more than nibble at the evergrowing problem. The success of this unit, however, helped to stimulate development elsewhere. Barnhill, whose name had been altered to Foresthall but which had changed little in other ways had become part of the National Health Service in 1948. The grossly unsatisfactory conditions under which patients were being treated there had been brought sharply to public attention. Professor Stanley Alstead, who succeeded Professor Morris as Regius Professor of Materia Medica, was in the vanguard of those who pressed for reform, and for the provision of scientific and humane treatment for the aged and chronic sick. The plight of many patients was vividly brought out by the early research work of two of Professor Alstead's staff, Dr (now Professor) John Brocklehurst and Dr Nanette Nisbet. In 1952 the Western Regional Hospital Board appointed Dr (now Professor) W. Ferguson Anderson to the new post of Consultant Physician at Foresthall and Regional Adviser on diseases of old age and chronic sickness. Thus began the organization of geriatric services in the City of Glasgow.

The problem which faced Dr Anderson was formidable. Geriatrics as a branch of general medicine was in its infancy, and had scarcely begun to be recognized. Few people had any clear idea of its function. The general physicians had expectations that the appointment of a geriatrician would mean that old people and the chronic sick would be taken care of by someone else, and that was about all. Where were the beds for geriatric patients to come from? Where were the doctors, the nurses and the ancillary workers? Virtually the only provision for geriatrics in the city was located in Foresthall, which was still little more than a Victorian poorhouse. To the public it was disgrace and degradation to enter its gates, and they held the conviction that 'you only came out in a box'. Foresthall had to be modernized, and medical, nursing, rehabilitation and social work staff of high calibre had to be attracted to it.

Dr Anderson's viewpoint was that the medicine of old age would, in future, assume a far more important place in the work of the medical profession. The only way to prepare doctors, nurses and ancillary staff for this new role was to locate geriatric admission units in general hospitals. He argued that ill old people admitted to hospital required the same facilities for investigation and medical treatment as ill people of any other age; only if they were investigated would the many opportunities for treatment which their illnesses afforded be identified and seized. This need of the ill old person for diagnosis and treatment was paramount, and long-stay wards must be reserved for patients who failed to benefit after a full trial of treatment in an admission ward.

With the assistance of the geriatric subcommittee of the Western Regional Hospital Board, Dr Anderson developed a plan under which the City of Glasgow and its environs was divided into five sectors, each based on one of the five major general hospitals in the city. Each sector had a population of about a quarter of a million. In each a geriatric unit was to be established in, or closely associated with, the general hospital, and this would be responsible for providing geriatric services for the local community and for the hospitals in the sector.

To implement this policy, beds, money and staff were required on an unprecedented scale. Initially many of the beds were obtained by taking advantage of medical and social change. Improved housing conditions, the introduction of antibiotics and a highly successful mass radiography campaign had enormously reduced the city's need for beds for tuberculosis and infectious diseases, and many of the beds thus released were seized upon and converted to geriatric use. The Regional Hospital Board scoured the city for undeveloped sites. A special financial allocation was made from central government funds, and new units of standard design were constructed wherever ground could be obtained. Nurses were attracted to working with old people, and many young doctors, observing the pace of development of the new speciality, saw in it the opportunities of a stimulating and satisfying career. The situation was not ideal.

Some buildings were structurally unsuited to the work that had to be done, some were inconveniently located, and some experienced shortages of staff and equipment. Outpatient and day-care facilities were insufficient. But an immense amount was achieved in a very short time, and by 1967, when the main survey was undertaken, Glasgow was fortunate in having an organized geriatric hospital service.

Parallel with the development of the geriatric service, a range of social services was provided by the Local Authority. In 1967 the Social Work (Scotland) Act had not yet been passed into law, and social services were organized by the Health and Welfare Department of the Corporation of Glasgow. The main services provided included residential care in old peoples' homes, the home help service, Meals-on-Wheels (in collaboration with the Women's Royal Voluntary Services), luncheon clubs, a district nursing service, domiciliary occupational therapy and home adaptation, chiropody (in association with the Red Cross), health visitors and visitation by social workers. All these services were available to the geriatric unit through the medical social work departments of the hospitals, but the supply fell short of the demand. A wide range of voluntary organizations provided various other services, and most of these were co-ordinated through the Glasgow Old Peoples' Welfare Committee.

In 1967 the geriatric unit, whose patients are to be described, had established a method of working and had acquired the basic facilities with which to perform the task. But much was still in a stage of evolution. The commitment of the unit was not clearly defined, old buildings were incomplete, and it operated against a background of shortages of beds, staff and ancillary services. There have been substantial improvements in all these respects since 1967, but demand has grown too, and geriatricians still struggle, as this unit did in 1967, to provide the best service consistent with limited resources.

The Department of Geriatric Medicine

Under the plan of the Western Regional Hospital Board the Department of Geriatric Medicine of Glasgow Royal Infirmary was established in 1964 to serve the needs of the eastern sector of the City of Glasgow. In 1966 and 1967 the new buildings of the department were not yet available and, when the survey was undertaken, the admission unit was located temporarily in a former infectious diseases hospital some miles away from the Royal Infirmary. In addition, the department had some 300 long-stay beds in five other hospitals.

The normal mode of operation of the unit was as follows. Patients

13

were referred to the department by general practitioners from the East End of the city and from the wards of Glasgow Royal Infirmary and its associated hospitals. Immediately after notification to the department, every patient was visited in his own home or in the hospital ward from which he was referred, by one of the two consultant geriatricians. At this visit a medical and social assessment was made, and a decision was taken on whether the patient should be admitted to the geriatric unit, referred to some other service or cared for at home.

Admission or transfer to the geriatric unit was recommended for patients with physical disease or disability who required the facilities of the unit, whether or not their illness was accompanied by mental symptoms or social problems. Referral to the psychiatric unit was advised for patients who were not apparently physically ill but who had prominent mental symptoms. Residential care was recommended for subjects who were not physically ill, or who had only a stable disability of moderate severity and known cause, but who required care and attention.

For patients not in need of hospitalization, advice on management was given to general practitioners, supplemented when appropriate by outpatient investigation. Patients were also put in touch with home helps, district nurses, Meals-on-Wheels, and a home-visiting service, or were offered a convalescent holiday, domiciliary physiotherapy, domiciliary occupational therapy, speech therapy or chiropody. For patients with stable disability who were being cared for at home short-term hospital admission was arranged during relatives' holidays.

Patients admitted to the geriatric unit underwent full medical and social investigation and rehabilitation. Those who recovered or improved sufficiently were discharged, and followed up at home. Those who had no adequate homes to return to but who were capable of self-care were referred to residential homes. Those who were too disabled to return to the community were transferred to the long-stay wards of the geriatric department where most of them stayed until they died, although a few improved and were discharged.

Figures relating to the working of the unit are given in Table 4 (p. 128). About two-thirds of the patients referred to the unit were accepted for admission. The number of accepted cases always exceeded the number of vacancies, and many patients had to wait up to four weeks or even longer before a bed became available. In that time some 10 per cent of the patients died, and another 5 per cent were admitted to other hospitals. One-third of the patients admitted to the geriatric unit improved sufficiently to be able to return home, usually after a stay of from one to three months. One-third died within three months of admission, and the remaining

14

one-third were transferred to long-stay wards after a stay of from one to three months in the admission ward. The average survival of patients in long-stay wards was about two years, although a few remained for upwards of five or even ten years. The average period of occupancy of a bed in the geriatric unit was just over six months. In other words, each bed in the geriatric unit was used to treat only two patients a year.

The majority of patients transferred from general medical and surgical wards failed to improve after full investigation and treatment, and, while some responded favourably to the intensive rehabilitation which they underwent in the geriatric unit, a substantial proportion became long-stay patients.

4 The Hard Core

What is geriatrics? Is it really a branch of medicine in its own right? Is there such a thing as a geriatric patient? Are special units needed to look after old people, or is this merely a convenient arrangement for preventing the beds in acute medical wards from being blocked by patients for whom nothing more can be done? Is it true to say that every general physician is in a sense a geriatrician? And if geriatrics is a speciality, what is its proper field?

These questions are widely debated in the medical profession. It is the conviction of all who work in the geriatric field that theirs is a specialty. They believe that the patients under their care are quite different from the majority of older patients in general medical wards; that they present peculiar problems of great complexity; and that special knowledge, skill and insight are required of a doctor who devotes himself to their care. The geriatrician thinks of himself as a true general physician who is concerned with the total management of his patient.

The main material on which this and the next few chapters are based is a survey of 612 patients referred to the geriatric unit, and the methods and results are given in detail in Part II. As a first step we tried to see what we could learn about geriatric patients by comparing four groups of old people. One was a series of patients aged sixty-five and over, accepted for admission to the geriatric unit. The second consisted of patients, also aged sixty-five and over, drawn from the same area in the eastern sector of Glasgow, who were admitted to the acute medical wards of Glasgow Royal Infirmary. These two groups were compared with one another in respect of their ages and of certain social and medical characteristics. They were also compared with the population as a whole, as enumerated in the 10 per cent sample census of 1966, and with a control group, drawn at random from the elderly population who were matched for age and sex with the geriatric patients.

The first finding to emerge from this comparison was that, although all the patients in the first two groups were aged sixty-five or over, there was a striking difference in age between the medical and the geriatric patients. Two-thirds of the medical patients were under the age of seventy-five, while more than two-thirds of the geriatric patients were aged seventy-five years or over. Only 1 in 30 of the medical patients was aged eighty-five or over, compared with 1 in 5 of the geriatric patients. In the population as a whole two-thirds of those aged sixty-five and over were under the age of seventy-five and only 1 in 20 was aged eighty-five and over. In their age distribution elderly medical patients were thus representative of the population as a whole, but geriatric patients were drawn predominantly from the oldest stratum of the community. In a word, elderly medical patients were young old people; geriatric patients were old old people.

The elderly medical patients were found to differ from the geriatric patients in other qualities. Of the medical patients, 40 per cent had a husband or wife alive, twice as many as among the geriatric patients. The difference was due only in part to the greater age of the geriatric patients, since comparison with the control group showed that there was a tendency for geriatric patients to be selectively drawn from the single and the widowed. Other social factors which distinguished the geriatric patients from medical patients were that more geriatric patients lived alone, more were poorly housed and more came from the lower social classes. Most of these differences were quite small, and some did not reach the level of statistical significance. The situation could be summarized by the statement that geriatric patients were older and more socially disadvantaged than elderly medical patients, but that the social factors were insufficient in themselves to account for the difference between the two groups.

Where then did the main difference lie? We turned to consider what happened when an old person took ill. The general practitioner was summoned, and it was he who decided whether to keep the patient at home, to send him into a general medical ward, or to seek his admission to the geriatric unit. What clinical factors influenced the family doctor in making this decision? From experience we postulated that patients who had been ill for a long time, with symptoms which created dependency on others, were those most likely to be referred to a geriatric unit; those with an illness of short duration, presenting a more 'acute' clinical picture, were more likely to be referred to a general medical unit. In pursuit of this hypothesis five symptoms, all characterized by dependency on others, were defined, and their presence and duration before admission were determined in the two groups of patients. The five symptoms

17

were: stroke, falls, inability to walk without human support from bed to toilet, incontinence, and severe mental abnormality—usually confusion or dementia. The definitions used are given in Part II of this book, and the results in Tables 17 to 20 (pp. 136-8).

Stroke occurred with equal frequency in the two groups of patients, but the other four symptoms were very much more common and of much longer duration in the geriatric than in the elderly medical patients. Three times as many geriatric as medical patients had a history of falls; five times as many geriatric patients were unable to walk at the time of their admission to hospital; and six times as many were incontinent. Only 5 per cent of the medical patients had mental abnormality, compared with almost 50 per cent of the geriatric patients. Two-thirds of the geriatric patients had two or more of these five symptoms of dependency; two-thirds of the medical patients had none of them.

The two groups also differed greatly in the duration of dependency. One-quarter of the geriatric patients had required nursing help and supervision at home for one year or longer before their referral to hospital, and three-fifths had required such care for more than a month. But only one-tenth of the medical patients had required help for more than one week before their admission.

Finally, the outcome of hospital treatment was compared in the two groups. There was a high early mortality in both sets of patients —rather higher in the geriatric than in the medical patients. Of medical patients who survived, the majority were discharged home rapidly, and three months after admission only 4 per cent were still in hospital. (Most of these had been transferred to the geriatric unit.) Of the patients admitted to the geriatric ward, less than one-third were discharged home within three months, one-third died, and the rest remained in hospital as long-stay patients until their death months or even years later.

The fate of the patients was related to their presenting symptoms. Especially was it noted that patients with incontinence and/or mental abnormality were very unlikely to be discharged home, while patients with neither of these symptoms had a high probability of discharge. This was so, irrespective of the unit to which the patient was first admitted, although the majority of patients with these symptoms were in fact admitted to the geriatric unit.

In addition to patients referred to the geriatric unit from their own homes, the department also had to deal with patients who were admitted in the first instance as emergencies to acute medical or surgical wards in the general hospital, and who were subsequently referred by the doctor in charge to the geriatric unit for further management. The medical and social characteristics of these patients are set out in Table 5 (pp. 128-9). They resembled closely the ordinary geriatric patients, and thus differed sharply from the general run of 'acute' medical patients. These appeared to represent a group of chronically dependent ill old people whose admission to hospital was precipitated by an episode of acute illness, necessitating immediate entry to a general unit. After treatment of the acute episode the underlying chronic problem remained, and help was sought from the geriatric unit. An example of the way in which the system worked was provided by an old lady who fell in circumstances very similar to those of Mrs McGoldrick. She was sent to hospital for an X-ray, and was found to have sustained a crack fracture of her femur, not requiring surgical treatment. But because a bone was broken she was admitted to an orthopaedic ward and only later referred from there to the geriatric unit.

A further small group of patients referred to the geriatric unit in the main survey was made up of those under the age of sixty-five. Half of these came from home and half from hospital; their characteristics are described in Table 6 (pp. 129-30). A few of these had acute illnesses, such as a recent stroke, for which the rehabilitation facilities of the geriatric unit were in demand. The majority were cases of chronic neurological disorder, no longer manageable at home, for whom the geriatric unit provided the only alternative to a hospital for the 'young chronic sick'. Under legislation passed since 1967, young chronic sick patients are not deemed suitable for admission to geriatric units, but neither then nor at the time of writing were sufficient beds available for them in special units within acceptable distances from their homes.

Almost one-half of the patients accepted for admission to the geriatric unit suffered from significant mental abnormality, usually a confusional state or dementia. A further seventeen patients from home and four from hospital with prominent mental symptoms who were referred for consideration by the geriatrician were not accepted for the geriatric unit but were passed on to a psychiatric hospital. The distinguishing feature of these patients was the absence of overt physical illness. It is the belief of the geriatric physician that in the majority of cases of elderly people with disturbed mental function the mental symptoms are caused, aggravated or accompanied by physical disease, and that in some of these cases the mental symptoms are abolished or relieved by treatment of the physical disease. The presence of mental symptoms is therefore no barrier to the admission of an elderly patient to a geriatric unit; on the contrary, it is often an indication of the patient's need for investigation and rehabilitation. The group of patients who were not accepted for the geriatric unit were apparently physically well, but severely demented. They had gross disturbances of behaviour, most notably a marked tendency to wander, which made it difficult for

19

them to be managed in a geriatric ward. The need for physical investigation of these patients remained, but this required to be undertaken in a psychiatric ward. Some of the characteristics of this group of patients are given in Table 7 (p. 130-1).

These findings support our hypothesis of the origin of geriatric patients. Ill old people present to their general practitioners one of two 'images'. If the patient is comparatively young, better off socially, recently taken ill, free from prominent symptoms of dependency and thought likely to return home after a short spell of hospital treatment, he will be referred to a medical unit. If he presents with the opposite 'image' of advanced old age, social deprivation, prolonged dependency and poor prospects of hospital discharge, he is labelled 'geriatric'. Geriatric patients form the 'hard core' of ill old people. Older than the old and more ill than the ill, they have been excluded from the main stream of medical care, and a whole parallel system has had to be constructed around their needs.

This situation can perhaps be better understood by borrowing from mathematics the concept of 'sets', and by illustrating this by what are known as Venn diagrams. In Figure 1(a) the square represents 'the set of all ill people' and the clear circle within it, Figure 1(b), is 'the set of all ill old people'. Within this, Figure 1(c), a smaller black circle has been drawn to represent the 'hard core', that is 'the set of severely incapacitated socially disadvantaged very old people'. The two circles in Figures 1(d) and 1(e) represent respectively 'the set of all patients in medical wards' and 'the set of all patients in geriatric wards'. In Figure 1(f) the two diagrams have been superimposed. The patients in the medical wards are mostly young; a proportion of them are drawn from 'the set of ill old people', but only a very few from the 'hard core' are included. Patients in the geriatric wards are drawn to only a very limited extent from the young; most are old people, and a high proportion of these come from the 'hard core'. However, much of the area of 'the set of ill old people' and of the 'hard core' remain outside both circles. Some of these ill people are in psychiatric wards or other hospital facilities, not shown in the diagram for the sake of clarity, but the great majority remain undiagnosed outside the circles of institutional care. They are, in the current phrase, 'in the community', and we shall later see what their needs are there, and what care they receive.

Meantime, let us reflect a little on the hard core. The hard core is a black circle in the heart of the ageing population. It is growing rapidly as the number of people who survive into advanced old age grows; as they outlive their spouses and friends; as their economic and social resources dwindle; and as the strength of their bodies and the clarity of their minds become eroded by undiagnosed

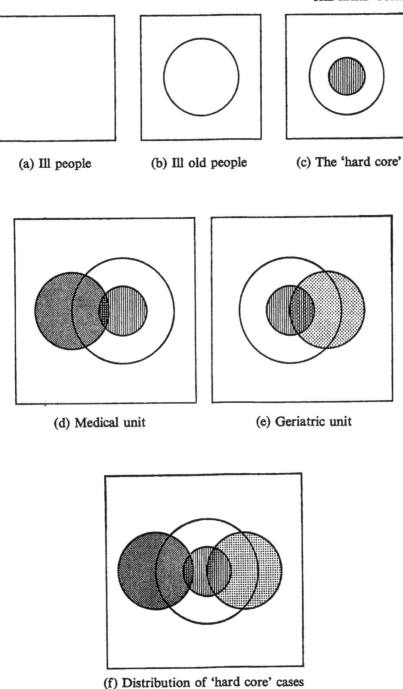

(a) Ill people   (b) Ill old people   (c) The 'hard core'

(d) Medical unit   (e) Geriatric unit

(f) Distribution of 'hard core' cases

Figure 1   Concept of the 'hard core'

and untreated disease. Already the hard core casts its black shadow over the health services, creating unprecedented and still growing demands for domiciliary and institutional care. This leads to complaints of blocked beds in general hospitals, overcrowding in mental hospitals and swelling waiting lists in geriatric units. If strangulation of services is to be avoided the growth of the hard core must be arrested; this can only be achieved by thoughtful, constructive action in which all branches of the health services must play a part. Geriatricians like Professor Anderson and Dr Nairn Cowan in Rutherglen and Dr J. Williamson and his colleagues in Edinburgh have shown that much can be done to prevent the formation of a hard core by reorganizing methods of medical care. Ill old people can be brought under observation at an earlier stage of their illness by using screening methods and early diagnosis clinics, and some apparently irreversible diseases can be ameliorated or eliminated by nothing more esoteric than the application of the accepted principles of medical diagnosis and treatment. The hard core is a threat to all. It should also be a challenge to all and a responsibility of all.

We commenced this chapter by asking, 'What is geriatrics?' Geriatrics is *not* the medicine of the hard core, but it might be defined as the method practised by doctors who are conversant with the problem of the hard core. The sceptic might define geriatrics as the treatment of underprivileged patients by underprivileged doctors, or we might borrow J. K. Galbraith's definition of politics and describe geriatrics as the choice between the impossible and the unpalatable. Whatever definition we favour, arresting the growth of the hard core must now become a major objective of the Health Service, and the geriatrician is the specialist best qualified to show how this can be done.

5　The Co-ordinates of Care

Doctors are accustomed to asking themselves the question, 'Why is this patient consulting me at this time about this illness?' When this question was asked about the patients who were referred to the geriatric unit, four main answers emerged. Either the patients were thought likely to be restored to a substantial measure of health by hospital treatment; or there was urgent medical need of admission, even although the eventual outcome appeared unfavourable; or the patient's immediate problem was lack of basic care at home; or else there was a threatened breakdown in the system of family care.

Of the 612 patients in the main survey 280 were referred from their own homes and were accepted for admission to the geriatric unit. These 280 patients were classified into four groups according to the answers to four questions which the doctor and the social worker asked themselves (see Figure 2).

1. Is it likely that the patient can be treated in hospital and discharged home again within three months?
   If the answer to this question was YES the patient was accepted for admission under the heading 'therapeutic optimism'. If the answer was NO the second question was asked.
2. Does the patient urgently need hospitalization for medical reasons, even though the prospect of discharge is poor?
   If the answer was YES the patient was admitted for 'medical urgency'. If the answer was NO the third question was asked.
3. Does the patient fail to receive adequate basic care at home; that is does he lack food, warmth, cleanliness or safety, as a result of his illness?
   If the answer was YES the patient was admitted for 'basic care': if NO, the fourth question was asked.
4. Are the patient's helpers suffering undue strain in caring for him? Undue strain was defined as a state of physical or mental

exhaustion created by the patient's illness.

If the answer was YES the patient was admitted for 'relief of strain'; if NO, the patient was not admitted.

The answers to these questions are given in Tables 8 to 11 (pp. 131-3).

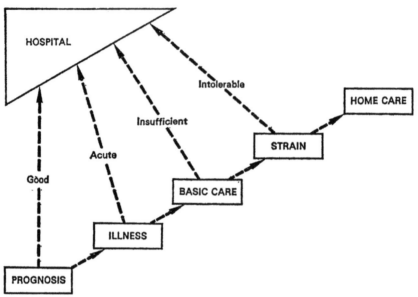

Figure 2 Reasons for acceptance to the geriatric unit

Fewer than one-half of the patients were accepted for primarily medical reasons—therapeutic optimism or medical urgency. More than one-half were admitted because of the social consequences of their illness, that is for the provision of basic care or the relief of strain.

'Therapeutic optimism' was the reason for admission of more than one-third of the cases. The optimism was justified in that one-half of this group were in fact discharged home within three months of their admission to the geriatric unit. As a group they were younger than the other geriatric patients, contained more who were married, more who had children in Glasgow, fewer who lived alone, and few who were incontinent. In their medical and social characteristics they were intermediate between the elderly patients admitted to general medical wards and the remainder of the geriatric patients. They contributed a great deal to the clinical interest of work in the geriatric wards, and the successful diagnosis and treatment of this group of cases was a major factor in the 'turnover' of patients in the geriatric unit. Examples of the type of patient admitted in this category included cases of stroke, acute respiratory disease and congestive

24

cardiac failure. In those cases in this group who additionally lacked basic care at home, or whose relatives were exposed to undue strain, successful treatment of the disease relieved the strain or abolished the need for basic care to be provided.

The group entitled 'medical urgency' was small and had a high mortality, since cases with a favourable prognosis were excluded from this category. Examples of this group included recent massive cerebral haemorrhage and advanced congestive cardiac failure.

The third group, those who were referred for admission because of 'insufficient basic care', accounted for one-quarter of all cases accepted from home. The reasons for these patients' failure to receive adequate basic care will be discussed in Chapters 6 to 9. Compared to the 'therapeutic optimism' group they were older, included fewer married subjects, more who lived alone, and more who had no children. Many had a history of falls, and many were mentally abnormal. In their duration of illness before referral they differed very little from the other geriatric patients. Only a few in this group were discharged home from the geriatric ward within three months of admission, and their early mortality was also low; as a result, more than half of the 'basic care' patients remained as long-stay cases.

The patients admitted primarily in order to relieve strain on relatives accounted for one-third of all the patients accepted for the unit. These patients received adequate basic care at home, were not especially in need of hospital treatment because of a medical emergency, and were thought to be unlikely to become fit for discharge. Indeed, only one-fifth of this group returned home within three months of admission to the geriatric unit. More than half of them died in that period, and the rest remained in hospital as long-term patients. Very many of these patients were bedfast, confused and incontinent at the time of their referral, and had been so for months or years previously. Few lived alone; the majority were with a spouse, a daughter or other close relative.

If the small 'medical urgency' group is excluded from the discussion, the geriatric patients in this series can be divided into three main groups according to the medical and social circumstances of their illness. First were the younger and socially better protected patients, for whom medical attention was sought at a stage when the illness was still amenable to treatment, and where favourable home circumstances allowed for planned discharge after treatment. Second came the socially isolated patients, who became gravely deprived of care when they were no longer able to look after themselves. Although they were the least ill of the three groups, their social resources were so poor that their restoration to the community was rarely possible, even after successful hospital treatment. The third group were well cared for at home by relatives who were reluctant to part with them until their illness reached such an advanced stage that the multiplicity of their needs could no longer be provided for at home. Their referral to hospital came in the final phase of their illness, and death followed soon after their admission to hospital.

The situation can be represented in the form of a diagram (Figure 3), using the principle of Cartesian paired co-ordinates. Every patient in the series can be looked upon as having a medical need for investigation and treatment, and a social need for the provision of basic and nursing care. If arbitrary scales of measurement of these needs were devised, each patient could be characterized by his position on these scales. In the diagram medical need is represented by the distance along the vertical axis and social need by the distance along the horizontal axis. If each case is plotted in this way the three main groups of patients appear as in the diagram: the 'therapeutic optimism' group is characterized by high medical and low social needs; the patients in the 'basic care' group have high social but low medical needs; and between them fall the 'strain' cases

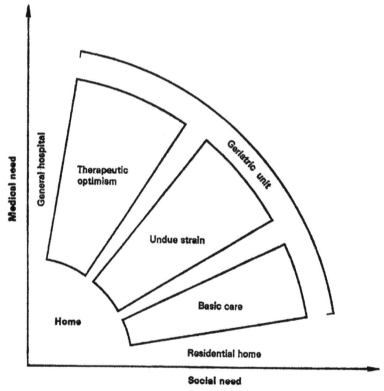

Figure 3   The spectrum of need

in whom both medical and social need are high. There are three empty spaces on the diagram: at the top is an area of high medical and low social needs which corresponds to acute medical cases; at the bottom are cases of low medical and high social needs, which are cases of old people who require re-housing, residential homes or domiciliary social services; the empty space near the origin refers to those many old people with comparatively modest medical and social needs lying latent in the community, who have not yet presented themselves for help from the geriatric service.

We may very well question whether our geriatric resources are being wisely used. Surely the function of a medical service is to treat medical need, and not to deal with the social consequences of unmet medical need. A complex of medical and social agencies should be marching into the unclaimed territory near the origin of the diagram, identifying and treating medical need while it is still of manageable proportions, supplying the social needs, and avoiding the disastrous consequences of unmet need. This indeed is the ideal, and this, or something resembling it, has been practised in many areas, using non-conventional methods of case-finding with encouraging results. However, this approach is not without its difficulties, as will be seen when we turn to consider what factors are responsible for the unmet needs of the aged sick.

6 Insufficient Basic Care

Throughout the main survey of 280 patients referred from their homes to the geriatric unit the expression 'insufficient basic care' was used to denote those cases where a patient failed to receive food, warmth, cleanliness and safety at the level at which he would have provided these for himself had he been fit to do so. Ninety-one cases were classified in this category, representing one-third of all the patients referred from home; in sixty-seven of these the patient's lack of basic care was the prime reason for his admission to the geriatric unit. These cases represented a partial or total breakdown of the system for providing for the weak and the needy. In the present chapter a description will be given of who these patients were and of what care they received or failed to receive. In the chapters which follow an attempt will be made to explain why they lacked care, and what might be done for them.

The following case report is an example of the circumstances in which an ill old man living alone failed to obtain sufficient basic care.

Mr Menzies, a bachelor and proprietor of a family grain business, lived alone in a large old-fashioned semi-detached villa in a quiet street, round which a Corporation housing estate had been built. At eighty-two he still went to his business every day, until he developed angina of such severity that he became housebound. His secretary came to the house with papers for him on two days a week, and he also received regular visits from a widowed niece, who was in full-time employment, an elderly couple—life-long family friends—and the clergyman who occupied the adjacent villa. He was also persuaded with great difficulty to agree to having a home help. Then one night he went down to the cellar to fetch coal, fell and was unable to rise. He lay all night unheeded until the home help found him cold and shocked next day. He was admitted to hospital where he did well and insisted on returning home. He was now much more shaky, but for some months this existence continued until one night his house was broken into by three young thugs. Gamely he tried to repel them, and was rewarded with a vicious beating-up. Once again he remained all night on the floor bruised and bleeding, until the arrival of the home help. He allowed himself to be taken to hospital to have his wounds dressed, but refused admission. For the next five months, until he finally consented to re-enter the geriatric unit, Mr Menzies lived in conditions of insufficient basic care. His gait and balance deteriorated so that he had difficulty in reaching the toilet, and frequently fell. He became incontinent and somewhat confused. He ate little. His gaunt house was damp and cold. His niece increased the frequency of her visits, his friend spent hours at a time in the house, the minister and his wife looked in whenever they could, the home help was loyal and devoted; but still there were long hours by day and night that this frail ill old man lay alone. Eventually after yet another fall he contracted a chest infection and consented at last to enter hospital, where he survived for only a few weeks.

Mr Menzies failed to receive, at an adequate level, all four of the ingredients of basic care. Food was supplied only intermittently; warmth he lacked because he was unable to stoke his fire; he lay for many hours in contact with his own excreta and thus lacked cleanliness; and he was ever in danger of falling with no one to help him and so lacked safety.

Of the ninety-one patients with 'insufficient basic care', twenty-seven including Mr Menzies lacked all four ingredients of care; but the majority lacked only two or three. No patient was without sufficient food or warmth alone, and all but one of those who lacked food and warmth also wanted for cleanliness or safety (see Table 31, p. 144). Presumably those old people in the community who had insufficient food or warmth, but who were clean and safe, were not ill enough to be referred to the geriatric unit. In the survey of geriatric patients 'insufficient basic care' nearly always meant that the patient was too ill to cleanse himself when he was soiled, or too weak in body or mind to protect himself from hazards, and that he was alone for much or all of the day or night.

Seventy-five of the ninety-one patients with insufficient basic care lacked safety. Most of these lacked safety because they were alone for long periods when they were in danger of falling and lying helplessly on the floor, but many others were unsafe because they tampered with gas, fire or electricity, or they wandered out into the streets at risk of being involved in traffic accidents. Here are examples of these.

Mrs Black was a widow of sixty-seven who suffered from Parkinson's disease. She lived alone in a single apartment with an outside toilet on the stairs, two floors up in an old tenement property. She had been housebound for ten years and could only walk about her little room slowly and unsteadily holding on to the furniture. Because of the tremor of her hands she could not hold a cup of tea. She would not admit to herself how disabled she was. She tried to do her own cooking and had fallen several times. Once she fell with a boiling kettle in her hands, but fortunately escaped injury. She had been warned not to attempt to rise from bed during the night if she needed the toilet and had been given incontinence pads and told to use them instead. The home help was willing to clean her in the morning, but the patient rarely used the pads, preferring to get up to the commode and take the risk of falling. Her only son lived some three miles away in a house with one room and a kitchen and an outside toilet. He had three children and his wife was expecting a fourth. They were saving up to buy a house and the son worked a lot of overtime. He visited the patient every evening, put her into bed, warned her not to get up, and went home worrying, knowing that no one would be in the house until the home help arrived the following morning. He told the social worker, 'This has been going on now for so long that I have forgotten what it is like to have peace of mind.' He had been called from his work on several previous occasions because the patient had been found lying on the floor by an elderly neighbour. She was eventually referred to the geriatric unit when she fell while attempting to return to bed after using the commode at night. She responded partially to rehabilitation, but was clearly unfit to return home, and was therefore transferred to a long-stay ward. Mrs Black, although stubborn, was mentally well. The lack of safety which surrounds a mentally abnormal patient is illustrated in the following example.

Mr Mackenzie, a widower of seventy-eight, lived with his divorced daughter in an attractively furnished Corporation flat. He was alone in the house all day while she was out at work. He had no other children and had quarrelled with his sister, herself old and frail and living at a distance, so that she rarely visited. He had a cardiac condition for which a pacemaker had been implanted, and he was also mildly demented; as his daughter said, 'There is no telling him.' Her main fear was fire, for Mr Mackenzie smoked his pipe incessantly, lighting it with strips of paper which he tore off newspapers, lit at the gas fire and threw, still burning, on to the carpet. But the tragedy which she had long dreaded came in a different way. One day Mr Mackenzie took it into his head to make himself a cup of tea. He turned on the oven instead of the gas tap but failed to appreciate his error. When the ring failed to light he turned on one of the other gas taps and lit it. The unlit gas from the oven seeped up and ignited. There was a terrific explosion. The oven door was blown off and shot across the room, the kettle hit the ceiling, and Mr Mackenzie was thrown on to his back, although he escaped serious injury. Terrified by the incident, the daughter could no longer cope and sought the patient's admission to hospital.

Many other mentally impaired patients endangered themselves and others through misuse of gas, fire or electricity, or by irresponsible behaviour in traffic. One set his clothing alight by standing too near an electric fire; several burned their pyjamas or bedclothes by smoking in bed; one electrocuted himself, not fatally, by poking a coal-effect electric fire; one fell into a real coal fire while poking it and sustained severe burns; one burned his legs by falling asleep in front of an electric fire; one old lady set her entire house on fire by her habit of piling up a tremendous amount of coal in a fireplace which was located immediately opposite the front door. There were countless incidents of demented patients burning out pots and kettles which had been left forgotten on the gas rings, and of gas escaping from cookers when they had been left unlit or extinguished by a pot boiling over. Once the doctor entered the house on a routine visit and found the patient lying unconscious in a gas-filled room; the tubing connecting the gas-poker to the supply had perished and the patient had failed to notice the smell of escaping gas. All these patients were repeatedly warned of the dangers, and many relatives installed fireguards, deprived the patient of matches, or turned the gas off at the main before leaving the house. But accidents continued to happen.

The next most frequent lack in this group of patients was that of cleanliness. Sixty-two subjects were unclean. Two-fifths of them were incontinent, and were habitually left in contact with urine or faeces, with no one available to change them. The others were continent, but through physical frailty, mental apathy and lack of help, they remained unwashed and allowed their houses to become filthy. The most appalling conditions were found in the homes of alcoholics, dements and recluses, especially among those who had known better days. Some were so ashamed of the dirt, food-waste and lumber with which they had surrounded themselves that they would not allow anyone to help clear up the mess, or even to cross the door. There were a few in this group who had accumulated legions of cats. Several had vast quantities of old newspapers piled on the floor, chairs and tables. Others specialized in pots, pans, china, glassware, jars and bottles—masses of them all over the floor. One elderly recluse was found in bed fully clothed, wearing two hats, one on top of the other, like a cricket umpire. In bed beside her she had twenty-two other hats. She also had nine cats in her filthy one-roomed house.

Lack of food and warmth were noted mainly in patients who also lacked cleanliness or safety, or both. The want of food was associated with isolation, apathy and frailty, and in some cases it reached a most lamentable extent. In one house the food cupboard stood empty; all that was to be seen were a loaf of bread, a packet of margarine, a pot of jam and a half-full bottle of milk turned sour on the kitchen table. In another, there were twelve tins of mushroom soup, but nothing else, not even a tin-opener. Another house boasted a dish on which were more than a dozen eggs, covered thickly with dust. The same dish, and doubtless the same eggs, were found when a follow-up visit was paid to the house several months later. Only two of the patients who lacked food received Meals-on-Wheels—few had even heard of the service. Twenty-two of them had a home help who gave them a meal when she came in and a cup of tea before she departed, and often left a flask of tea or a sandwich to be eaten later. But these patients had nothing else to eat or drink in the twenty-four hours. Many depended on food brought in by a neighbour or a daughter. One man with multiple sclerosis was given a meal by his unmarried son when he returned from his work in the evening, consisting usually of fish and chips brought in from a café, but the son went off to work in the morning without offering the patient a cup of tea or making provision for his midday meal. Another old man dying of cancer of the lung lived alone and was found in a state of near starvation, but he barred the door against his daughter-in-law when she came with food for him. Similar to him was a demented old lady living alone whose daughter-in-law brought food to her, and she then threw it out of the window.

Although emaciation and malnutrition were seen in this group of patients very few of them complained of hunger, but many felt the lack of something else. 'I lie here all day,' said one bed-bound lady with rheumatoid arthritis, 'and there's no one so much as to bring me a cup of tea.'

Lack of warmth was also found mainly in those living alone or with an elderly spouse only. One-half of the houses of those who were without sufficient warmth depended on coal fires entirely, and the physical difficulty of keeping the fire going was a major factor. Again home helps and neighbours helped a great deal, but could not provide all the help that was needed. Cost and apathy were other factors responsible for the patient receiving insufficient heat. Electric and gas heaters were, in the main, old-fashioned and inefficient in those houses which depended on them. Heat losses were excessive in some damp, draughty old tenement houses. Many patients were thinly clad or had inadequate bedclothes. Yet few of those who lacked warmth actually complained of cold, and no case of hypothermia was found.

In an attempt to identify who these ninety-one patients were who lacked adequate basic care a comparison was made between them and the 189 geriatric patients whose basic care was adequate (see Tables 21 and 32, pp. 139 and 145). The two groups differed little in age and sex, but those who lacked basic care were more socially isolated. Only 1 in 9 of them was married, and three-fifths had no children in the Glasgow area. Nearly two-thirds lived alone, and one-half dwelt in houses which lacked a bathroom. Only 1 in 5 had the services of a district nurse, but one-half of them had a home help. This was three times the proportion of those with 'sufficient care' who had a home help. The explanation of the relatively high utilization of home helps by those who lacked adequate basic care seemed to be that the home help had endeavoured to provide for the patient's twenty-four-hour needs during the course of her two- or four-hour stay, and had at least succeeded in maintaining the patient alive. This will be discussed more fully in Chapter 15.

The 'insufficient basic care' cases were, as a group, less ill than the others at the time of their acceptance for the geriatric unit. Fewer in the group had suffered a stroke, were immobile or were mentally abnormal; fewer had been dependent for more than one year before referral. The mortality rate in the first three months after admission to hospital was comparatively low for the 'insufficient basic care' patients, and so too was their discharge rate from hospital. As a result, one-half of them remained in hospital as long-stay patients. This was because the diseases from which they suffered and the social conditions from which they originated were alike insusceptible to radical treatment.

In the eastern area of Glasgow in 1967 a very substantial part of the demand for admission to the geriatric unit came from isolated ill old people who lacked adequate basic care.

7 The Anatomy of Neglect: Preoccupation

In the previous chapter we described ninety-one neglected old people living in a welfare state in conditions of filth, hunger, cold and danger, which no one could look upon without crying out for immediate action. Only a handful of these patients were wholly without help —the majority were assisted by relatives, friends, neighbours and the social services—but the help fell short, in some cases far short, of the patients' needs. Fifty-two of these unfortunates were alone, or almost alone, in the world, and the insufficiency of their care is comprehensible. They included eight bachelors, twelve spinsters, fourteen childless widows and four childless widowers; a further fourteen subjects were, for practical purposes, virtually childless since their children lived outside the Glasgow area. Help flowed to most of these people from grandchildren, nieces, sisters, cousins and other more distant family members, often at a cost of severe strain to the helpers. Neighbours and friends, too, were generous in their assistance, and home helps and district nurses visited and cared for several in the group. However, all this was not enough. Most of the patients who failed to receive sufficient basic care needed someone with them throughout the twenty-four hours, and it was this lack of continuous care which led to the unacceptable conditions in which they were referred to the geriatric service.

What of the thirty-nine patients in this group who did have children living in Glasgow? Surely it was the responsibility of the family to ensure that their parents were not allowed to remain in the state of insufficient care in which they were found? Were the children of these thirty-nine patients shirking their responsibilities and leaving it to the state to look after the old people, or were there other reasons for the apparent neglect? This was the question to which we now turned our attention.

The investigation in detail of these thirty-nine cases was undertaken by the social workers with particular care. Efforts were made to track down relatives and to overcome their hesitancy, reluctance or hostility. The social worker had to listen patiently to partial truths in the hope that the full truth would eventually emerge. Where more than one family member was involved she listened to every side of the story and pieced together her own assessment of where the truth lay. At weekly meetings her knowledge of the circumstances was presented and discussed with the doctor and the other social workers. Finally, each case was placed in one of four categories, which were called 'preoccupation', 'dilemma', 'refusal' and 'rejection'. The relationship between these categories is illustrated in Figure 4.

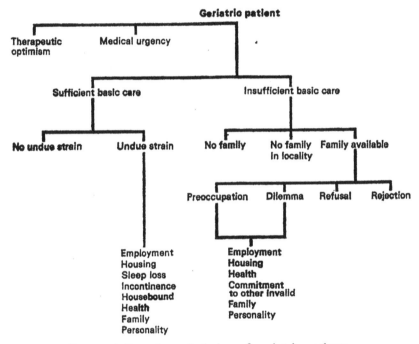

Figure 4   Factors influencing admission of geriatric patients

'Preoccupation' was considered to be the reason why seventeen of the thirty-nine patients with children in Glasgow failed to receive adequate care. The term was used to describe circumstances where relatives provided as much care as they could, and were anxious to give even more help, but were prevented from doing so by a prior commitment from which they were quite unable to free themselves, or by an impediment which they could not overcome. The following case is an example of lack of basic care due to 'preoccupation'.

35

Mrs Cormack, a widow of seventy-two, lived alone in a drab and cheerless but adequate Corporation house. She came to the door herself to answer the doctor's call, and stood for a while, blue-grey, gasping for breath, clad in a flannel nightgown and a man's coarse dressing-gown untied around her, and with bare and dirty feet. She shuffled her way painfully back to the bedroom, clutching on to the wall, and climbed into bed where she lay exhausted for some minutes before regaining sufficient breath to answer the doctor's questions. The house was untidy and smelt of stale urine. Mrs Cormack was partially paralysed as a result of a stroke four years previously. She also had heart disease and was subject to terrifying paroxysms of breathlessness at night, as well as to the breathlessness on exertion which the doctor had witnessed. She had great difficulty in reaching the toilet and thus often wet herself. Indeed, she had done so not long before the doctor's visit, as was unpleasantly obvious. She was a depressed, miserable, critical individual with never a kind word for anyone. When the doctor asked who there was to help her she replied that she had a daughter, 'but I might as well be dead for all she cares'. The facts proved to be very different. Mrs Cormack's only daughter, aged forty-nine, was married with one son of twelve, and lived at about fifteen minutes' walk from the patient. She was subject to asthmatic attacks. Ever since the death of the patient's husband nine years previously, the daughter had come every day to Mrs Cormack's house. She did the shopping, the washing, the cleaning and the cooking, while the patient offered criticism rather than appreciation. However, the daughter's husband, who had worked as a miner, was crippled with pneumoconiosis and, at about the time of Mrs Cormack's stroke, he had had to give up work. The daughter obtained employment as a school cleaner working from 6 till 8.30 a.m. and 4 till 6.30 p.m. daily. For the past year her twelve-year old son had slept in Mrs Cormack's house so that she should not be alone at night, as he was able to get himself out to school in the morning. The daughter's day (when she was not confined to her bed with an asthmatic attack) therefore began at 5 a.m. when she rose and made herself a cup of tea. She went out to her work, and on her way back called in at her mother's to see that all was well, to feed and change her and to make her son's bed. She then went home to tidy her own house, to look after her husband and to do the shopping for two households. She managed a second visit to the patient's house before returning to her work. On her way home from work, she paid her third visit to Mrs Cormack, made supper for her and for her son and settled them both for the night before returning home. She had suggested a home help to Mrs Cormack who had indignantly rejected the idea, 'What do I need with a home help when I have a daughter?' There would in any case have been a substantial charge for this service which would have been ill afforded, and Mrs Cormack refused to apply for social security benefits. This situation had continued until the day before the doctor's visit, when the daughter failed to turn up because she had contracted influenza. The daughter was more concerned about Mrs Cormack than about herself and had urged the family doctor to try to get her into hospital. That was why the geriatrician had been called to the house. This patient was unfit and unsafe to be left alone, and would not be adequately helped by the domiciliary services. She required admission to hospital but there was little probability of significant clinical improvement. She lacked basic care because of the daughter's 'preoccupation' with her own illness, the illness of her husband, her employment and the care of her own son.

In these cases of 'preoccupation', the factors responsible were classified as follows:

Health of helper	7 cases	Care of small children	2 cases
Health of another		Employment of helper	7 cases
dependant	6 cases	Lack of accommodation	4 cases

In the case of Mrs Cormack and in several others, more than one factor was present. Mrs Cormack's daughter could not continue to care for her because she was prostrated with a severe respiratory infection. Three other geriatric patients were suddenly left without basic care when their principal helpers became acutely ill and were admitted as emergencies to hospital. Three further patients depended on relatives barely capable of looking after themselves, far less an ailing patient. Of these one helper had rheumatoid arthritis, one had chronic bronchitis and one, the son of a confused old lady, was himself a schizophrenic on temporary discharge from a mental hospital. In these cases, as the patient grew more dependent the relatives were less and less able to cope, until the care provided became so inadequate that the patient had to be rescued by admission to hospital.

In six other cases the relatives were 'preoccupied' by the care of other ill people. One old woman, unfit to live alone because of a previous fracture of the femur, was left all night and visited only briefly during the day. She had two daughters in Glasgow, but each had one of her own husband's parents living with her who was unfit to be left alone; so the daughters had to wait until their husbands came in from work before they could visit the mother. There were two other cases of daughters with parents-in-law to look after, two with invalid husbands—one with a coronary and one dying of cancer—and one with a mentally and physically defective child who required constant attention.

Two patients with strokes, both in their early sixties, had daughters who were 'preoccupied' with the care of young children. This was a rare cause of 'preoccupation', because most of the patients were of an age when their daughters' families were grown up. One of the daughters had a large family, of whom three were under the age of three. The other daughter had an only child, a boy of six, born to her after sixteen years of marriage, when she had abandoned hope of ever becoming a mother, and, as she said, very dear to her. The patient, Mrs Weir, was bedfast, incontinent and helpless after suffering a hemiplegia four years previously. The patient's husband was himself an invalid with chronic bronchitis. His only contribution to Mrs Weir's care was to spit into the fire and to say, in a voice that brooked no contradiction, 'She's no' going into hospital!' This meant that Mrs Weir's daughter had to travel by two buses each way every day to and from her own house in a distant Corporation housing scheme. When the daughter was away her son would come home from school to an empty house or to the care of a neighbour. The daughter was unhappy about this arrangement. Her son was picking up words and habits in the neighbour's house of which she disapproved. He had started to wet the bed, and she had been called to see the headmaster because he had played truant from school. But she could not leave Mrs Weir. She told the social worker, 'I spend one-third of the day at my house worrying about my mother, one-third at my mother's worrying about my son, and one-third in the bus worrying about them both.'

There were seven patients who failed to receive adequate care because a son or daughter, who was willing and anxious to provide full care, was prevented from doing so by their employment. These seven comprised two unmarried sons, one unmarried daughter, one widowed daughter and three married daughters whose husbands were incapacitated. All these were sole wage earners. They justifiably feared that if they gave up their work they would be unable to find other employment again. They made such arrangements as they could to cover the patients' care during their necessary absence, but in these seven cases such arrangements were unavoidably insufficient to meet the patients' needs.

In four cases the housing situation was responsible for the patients' inadequate care. These were all ill old people living alone or with an aged spouse who were unfit to be on their own, and who could have received adequate care only if they had come to live with another family member. The relative in each case expressed an apparently genuine desire to have the patient in her house, but this was physically impossible because there was simply no room in the house. In three of these four cases the daughter's house consisted of one room and kitchen with an outside toilet and it already contained three or more people. The fourth daughter had a good three-bedroomed house, but this was already fully occupied by herself, her husband and their five children.

The following case is a further illustration of 'preoccupation'. Mr Daly, sixty-eight years of age, was found by the doctor lying flat on his back in bed like a plank of wood, quite unable to bend at the hips or knees, in considerable pain, and soiled with urine and faeces. Beside him was his elderly wife, bent double as she tried in vain to clean him up, apologizing for hurting him, but quite unable to lift him. Mr Daly had suffered from rheumatoid arthritis for twenty-six years, for the past ten of which he had been wholly confined to bed. His wife and daughter had nursed him and he had never been in hospital. His daughter married, but managed to rent a house in the same tenement as the patient. Then the tenement was scheduled for demolition, and both the patient and the daughter were re-housed—more than a mile away from each other. The daughter continued to spend almost every day helping to care for the patient, even long after she became pregnant. The geriatric service was contacted for help only when the daughter went into labour. He was then in great discomfort because his wife could not handle him alone, and there was no one else to help. He was obliged to pass faeces into the bed, although he had full control of his bowels.

The phenomenon of 'preoccupation' is a manifestation of the many demands which life can make on the middle-aged, the generation who are the sons and daughters of old people. Many in this generation are themselves at an age when their health and the health of their spouses is beginning to fail, and when commitments to their own children have not yet ceased. It is inevitable that 'preoccupation' will continue to prevent a proportion of otherwise willing relatives from caring adequately at home for the ill old people of the future.

8   The Anatomy of Neglect: Dilemma, Refusal

The cases of insufficient basic care to be described in this chapter include four where care was withheld because relatives, although capable and desirous of giving more help than they did, were forced to adopt a different course in the interests of their own families; and seven where help willingly offered by relatives was refused by the patients.

The four former cases were grouped under the heading 'dilemma' and came somewhere between 'preoccupation', where the relatives had virtually no choice, and the cases of 'rejection' to be described in the next chapter, where the relatives deliberately chose to withhold care. The dilemma of the children in these cases was whether to give prior consideration to the needs of the parent or to those of their own family. In the end they attempted to do both, and, as a result, the parent received insufficient basic care. This category was not easy to define, and therefore all four cases will be described. The descriptions can scarcely convey the tension, the anguish, the feelings of guilt which those caught in this cruel web of circumstance experienced over their decisions.

Mrs Colgan, a blind widow of seventy-seven, had been in hospital on many occasions with a bowel complaint, which was finally treated by colostomy. She also had a discharging abscess in her abdominal wall, which required frequent dressings. Because of her blindness she could not attend to herself and depended on the district nurse. She was arthritic and weak, and could not find her way about her house. She blundered into the furniture and was terrified of falling. At the time of the doctor's visit in the evening, Mrs Colgan's son was in the house. He was so obviously concerned and had such a good relationship with the patient that the doctor asked him if it was not possible for Mrs Colgan to go to stay with him. His reply was evasive, so it was left to the social worker to explore the situation.

She visited the son's home, a beautiful bungalow in a good residential area. The son was perfectly frank. 'I'll do as much as I possibly can for my mother', he said. 'Already I visit her for three hours every evening, and my wife goes twice a week. We have a private domestic help for her whom we pay, and we have advertised for someone to stay with her at nights, but have had no suitable replies. I can hardly sleep worrying about her living alone. I have even offered to put her in a nursing home, but she refuses. But I am afraid I cannot take her here.' He explained that his wife was extremely and obsessively fastidious. He had had the patient staying with him for a few months. The smell of the colostomy, the pus from the abscess and the soiled dressings to be disposed of had sickened his wife. She had gone about the house throwing open the windows, squirting deodorants and spraying antiseptics everywhere. 'I know that nurses have to put up with much worse,' said the son, 'but my wife is not made that way, and I have to live with her and consider her.' Furthermore, Mr Colgan's own teenage children had had to give up the room where they entertained their friends, and indeed were convinced that their friends no longer came to the house because of the smells and the draughts. 'You can't expect them to understand,' said Mr Colgan, 'they're only young.' And so Mr Colgan had chosen. His wife and family came first. He would do his best for his mother, but not at the cost of disrupting his own family life any further. As a result, Mrs Colgan was admitted to the geriatric unit for provision of basic care.

The second case was somewhat similar. Mrs Stewart, an old lady of seventy-nine, lived alone in an adequate but dreary flat. She was ambulant but depressed, mildly demented and incontinent. She was visited daily by her daughter who washed her, changed her, gave her meals and tidied the house, but seemed to do so coldly and resentfully. When the social worker visited the daughter in her exquisite home in a fashionable suburb, she was surprised by her insight and objectivity. The daughter described the life-long inadequacies of Mrs Stewart as a wife, mother and housekeeper, explained how she had escaped from the deadening influence, taken a job as a secretary, married well and risen in the social scale. 'My mother and I have nothing in common,' she said, 'but I will not neglect her.' When Mrs Stewart had first shown evidence, two years previously, of physical and mental deterioration, she had come to stay with the daughter. She had been unhappy there, envious of the daughter's wealth and resentful of her way of life. She took to standing at the garden gate, button-holing passers-by, and telling them how unhappy she was and how cruel her daughter was to her. There were frequent rows, and it was by mutual agreement that Mrs Stewart returned to her own flat, and to the conditions of inadequate basic care which led to her referral.

The third patient was again a blind old widow of seventy-five, who never adapted to her blindness, became depressed and excessively irritable. The patient talked incessantly, bemoaned her fate, criticized her relatives and demanded attention. She asked for a drink of water eight times and for a bed-pan three times in the course of the fifteen minutes that the doctor spent in the house. Her daughter-in-law was wonderfully patient. She was extremely upset at the old lady being left alone, and she was prepared to help as much as possible, but about one thing she was quite clear. 'I'm not having her in my house, and that's flat,' she said. 'She would have all of us in the mad-house.' One could not but agree.

Mrs Miller, also a seventy-five-year old widow, was confined to bed with cerebral arteriosclerosis and was incontinent. She received only one visit a week from her daughter, and for the rest of the time depended on the willing but none too efficient attentions of an elderly male lodger. The daughter did not work and lived only twenty minutes away. She did a great deal for the patient during her weekly visit and was obviously concerned about her, and the doctor failed to discover why she did not come more often. The social worker found the reason—the daughter had a Mongol daughter, now herself aged eighteen, and had never overcome her feelings of shame and guilt. She would not allow the girl to be left on her own, would not take her out with her, and entrusted her to no one except her husband. He worked a great deal of overtime, and it was only rarely that Mrs Miller received the attention which her daughter would gladly have given more often had not her dilemma prevented her.

In these four cases did the relatives make the right choice? Might they have chosen differently if there had been no geriatric service available to care for their parents? Each reader will have his own answer to these questions. By the time the geriatrician was called in to visit, the decision had already been taken. In no case had it been an easy decision for the family to take. Complex situations of the kind described as 'dilemma' will always exist. Amongst the 280 geriatric patients there were only four in this category. We do not know how many others, faced with similar agonizing choices, decided not to summon help from the geriatric service.

Let us turn now to look at the seven patients who lacked adequate basic care because of their own refusal to accept willing offers of help from relatives. Six of these seven patients were men. Four of the men and the one woman had a common personality type. They had always been aggressively independent. They had little love for others and attracted little towards themselves. They would not admit to themselves that they needed help, and would not put themselves in a position of being obliged to anyone else. The woman had quarrelled violently with her two sons when they took what she considered to be unsuitable wives, and wanted nothing further to do with them. When she fell and fractured her femur her sons and her daughters-in-law came to help her, but she would not let them in and shouted through the door that she neither wanted nor needed them.

These five patients were found in dreadful conditions of deprivation. They were truculent, uncommunicative or aggressive, and it was not always possible for the doctor or the social worker to penetrate to the roots of their self-hatred. How, for example, was one to interpret a situation when a widower of seventy-eight, half-crazed and dying of bronchial carcinoma, living in a filthy, unheated, ramshackle room, barred the door against his own son who lived in the same tenement, would not allow him or his wife access in case, as he said, 'they messed the place up', and only grudgingly accepted a hot cooked meal handed round the corner of the door? Or what was to be made of a man of eighty-two who left hospital against medical advice, refused to go and stay with his daughter who was willing to have him, and insisted on living alone, although he was desperately breathless, alarmingly unsteady on his feet, barely able to walk, and incontinent, and well knew that his daughter, who lived several miles away and had a young family, could not manage to visit him more than twice a week?

Another man of eighty-three lived with his wife and three sons, one daughter-in-law and several grandchildren, but he would allow no one except his wife to attend to him. He was enormously obese, coarse-featured, unkempt and deaf, with a fearful temper which he vented ceaselessly on his wife. He had a huge hernia which rendered it almost impossible for him to pass urine, and when he required to do so he roared like an angry bull for his wife, physically assaulting anyone else who tried to come to his aid.

In another case, a widower of seventy-eight was found living with a bachelor brother in conditions so deplorable that the sight and the smell linger long in the memory. The patient, who had advanced heart disease, died within hours of his admission to the geriatric unit. At first he was thought to have had no other family, but a daughter arrived at the hospital to claim the death certificate. She explained that many years previously the patient had deserted his wife and eight children in Ireland, and had drifted to Glasgow. One of his daughters subsequently married, came with her husband to live in Glasgow and encountered the patient purely by chance. Finding him ill and helpless she and her husband had repeatedly offered to take him to stay with them or to allow her to nurse him, but the patient, no doubt consumed by remorse and self-hatred, had angrily repulsed her aid.

Of the two patients whose refusal to accept help was not due to self-hatred, one was a widower of sixty-eight, the mildest of men, who was very fond of his only daughter, but firmly believed that young people should be free to live their own lives unfettered by the aged. When he became arteriosclerotic, incontinent, mildly confused and incapable of caring for himself, he would not go to stay with her. The other was a man of seventy-four who suffered a stroke two weeks after the death of his wife. He was admitted to a general hospital but left against medical advice before he was fit to do so. His daughter begged him to stay with her, but he refused because, as he said, 'I must work things out for myself.' He was quite incapable of looking after himself and it was impossible for his daughter to be with him all the time. He was referred to the geriatric unit for further hospital care.

The majority of the patients who refused help were thus motivated by feelings of self-hatred or aggression to pretend to themselves that their health was intact and that they had no needs. They violently refused offers of help because they would not allow their sons or daughters, against whom they had aggressive feelings, to assume a role of kindliness towards them. They refused help also from home helps and hospital nurses, whom they must have conceived of as a sort of 'daughter substitute'. To care adequately and early for strange patients like these must lie for ever beyond the wit of the welfare state, but fortunately their number is few.

9 The Anatomy of Neglect: Rejection

Eleven patients with insufficient basic care remain to be considered. All were found in abominable conditions of filth and neglect. All were ill and badly in need of care. All had children in the Glasgow area who were capable of extending help to them, but who refused to do so. The initial impression obtained was that these patients were heartlessly and selfishly neglected by their own flesh and blood. But was this truly how things stood? The following three cases, typical of this group, provide the answer.

Mr Tuckett, a widower of seventy-eight, was found living alone in appalling conditions of filth. He was confined to bed and doubly incontinent. He had an old fracture of the femur, as a consequence of which he could walk only with difficulty, and he suffered from malnutrition, but he had no other obvious disease. He refused to enter hospital, and his compulsory admission had to be arranged by application to the Court. Of his three children only one, a daughter, lived in the Glasgow area. When she was interviewed in her comfortable bungalow by the social worker, she was initially sullen and hostile, but after a few minutes she burst into tears, begged the social worker to sit down, gave her a cup of tea and poured out her story. The patient, it appeared, had been a civil engineer in an excellent position, with a nice house, a good wife and three children. Then he had taken to drink, and the daughter recalled with horror his drunken homecomings, his terrifying rages, her mother's endless struggles against unpaid bills, the impounding of furniture. The children left home as soon as possible—the sons to join the army, the daughter to take jobs which led to her early and happy marriage. As long as her mother remained alive, she paid occasional visits to Mr Tuckett, now pitifully sunk in the social scale. After her mother's death she lived in dread of her father's arrival at her door claiming to have reformed, begging for another chance. She had taken him in in the past, and given him clothes, food, shelter and money, but each time the reformation was brief, he started drinking again, shamed the daughter and her husband in front of their friends, terrified the children, insulted his son-in-law and eventually was put out. After years of misery she still felt guilty at the withering of her love for her father. She said to the social worker, 'I know it is wicked of me to say this, but I beg of you, please tell the doctor that I can't, I just can't ever again have him in my house. If I even start visiting him he will worm his way round me. He is cleverer than I am, I know.'

In the next case, when the doctor called, the door was opened to him after some delay by a shambling, shaggy, watery-eyed little man, who unsteadily led the way into the patient's room. Although it was broad daylight, the windows were shuttered and the room was lit by a naked bulb. The room was absolutely bare except for a double bed and a small bedside table. In the bed, from which the shaggy man had recently risen and to which he now returned, was the patient—a pale, thin woman, breathless, and fully dressed. At the bedside was a bottle of British sherry which she and her paramour were sharing. The doctor was most hospitably invited to join the party. The poor woman was dying of anaemia, and, indeed, died soon after her admission to the geriatric unit. On a crushed piece of paper she had the address of a daughter. Later the social worker visited this daughter and sought information on the patient's background. Her story was that the patient had been drinking for thirty years, had left her husband and home, had taken up with various shady men, had lived in a great variety of squalid rooms, such as the sub-let in which she was found, and had served numerous terms in prison for various petty offences. She descended on her three children at lengthy intervals, when all other sources of drinking money had dried up. They were all respectable working people, and viewed the patient with horror and loathing. They frankly admitted that they were not prepared to lift a finger to help her. One of them expressed her attitude in a not inappropriate cliché, 'She has made her own bed, let her lie on it.'

Alcohol was also a factor in the life of Mrs Duncannon, a poor crazed crippled woman who opened the door to the doctor after literally crawling from her bed on her hands and knees. This had been her sole method of locomotion for twelve years, and her inability to move about in any other way than this was a consequence of tabes dorsalis, one of the late manifestations of syphilis, the heritage of her career as a prostitute. Her youngest daughter lived in Glasgow but rarely visited, and her only assistance came from a home help and a gentleman friend. The daughter was interviewed by the social worker. She was at first reticent, but then broke down and told the social worker a lurid story of her childhood with the patient in the Glasgow slums. She had no father, only a succession of 'uncles'. She never remembered being warm, well-fed or comfortable, or of receiving any affection. She was eventually taken away from 'home' by the Welfare Department to work as a maid-servant on a Highland farm. She later married happily, settled in Glasgow, made tentative gestures of help towards the patient, succeeded partially in convincing herself that her help was not wanted, and almost succeeded in suppressing awareness of her mother's existence. In this her older brothers and sisters were more successful, because they had not visited since they had been taken away from home as children. The daughter who was interviewed still had residual feelings of guilt, which she expressed to the social worker in the words, 'Well you know, your mother's your mother; you can't help it in spite of what she is.'

There were four other cases in this group of long-standing family breakdown and social degradation in which alcohol played a major role. In none of these cases had the old person been a true parent. The family had grown up in poverty, accustomed to being roared at or beaten by a drunken father, to watching parents quarrel and strike one another, to seeing the furniture pawned, and to going hungry and unclad because of the parent's degradation. There had never been love between parent and child, but the son or daughter nearly always experienced a residual feeling of duty, which prompted an occasional generous act or a stirring of guilt. The parent was quick to exploit any gestures of kindness made towards him, with characteristically disruptive effects on the life of the son or daughter.

In two other of the eleven cases the rejection of a mother by the children was traced back, not to alcohol, but to a bitterly resented second marriage, since when all contact between parents and children had ceased. In each case the patient's second husband had children of his own, and the attitude of the patient's own children was 'let them look after her'. In the two remaining cases neither alcohol, crime, prostitution nor a second marriage could be invoked as an excuse for the children's behaviour. One of the patients was a widow of eighty-five, the other of eighty-nine. Both lived alone, neglected by families who might have helped; both had lived loveless lives and had roused discord, strife and dissension amongst their families, playing one off against another, criticizing, interfering and harassing. Now both were left unloved and uncared for by well-to-do selfish children who had never been brought up to sacrifice present comfort for the sake of conscience. In both cases the sons made a great play of visiting the patients in hospital, but were not prepared to make more than a token effort to provide help at home.

These eleven cases were classified under the heading 'rejection' because of the relatives' failure to provide adequate basic care.

47

Rejection there was indeed, but it must be remembered that it was the parents who rejected the children long before the children rejected the parents.

The findings detailed in the last four chapters may now be summarized. Among a consecutive series of 280 geriatric patients no fewer than ninety-one, or one-third, lacked adequate basic care at home at the time of their referral. Of perhaps two of these (less than 1 per cent of the entire group) might it justifiably be said that they had to enter hospital because their families were not prepared to do anything to help them. Seven others who received no help from their families (comprising $2\frac{1}{2}$ per cent of the series) were recruited from amongst the drunks, prostitutes and criminals of society, and had effectively cut themselves off from their children long before they reached old age. Two others had broken with their families over a disputed second marriage, and were considered to have abdicated their position as parents. To these eleven patients (4 per cent of the series) might be added another seven who reacted to long-standing family breakdown and personality abnormalities by refusing to accept help; while there were another four patients whose relatives, faced with what was admittedly a most difficult dilemma, decided that the needs of the elderly parent had to be subordinated to the family's other needs. Thus the number of patients whose lack of basic care could in any way be attributed to the negligence of the family varied from two to twenty-two, depending on one's criteria; that is from less than 1 per cent to, at very most, 8 per cent of the patients who required admission to the geriatric unit. In the other sixty-nine cases where patients lacked basic care the cause was either that they had no children, or that the children were so unavoidably preoccupied by other cares as to be incapable of providing the necessary assistance. In the present study neglect of parents by children was rare: failure of children to accept their responsibilities played only a negligible role in the demand for geriatric hospital accommodation. But the long-term effects of social inadequacy were all too evident. The childless young became the childless old; the aged alcoholic had all the problems of the young alcoholic; the misfits of years gone by were still misfits at the end of their days.

Not only did patients who lacked basic care at home comprise a high proportion of those who entered hospital but they also contributed a major share to the pool of long-stay hospital patients. Nearly one-half of them were still in hospital one year after admission, and many might be expected to survive for several years, without ever becoming fit to live outside hospital. If vital hospital beds are to be freed for use by other patients it is desirable that basic care should be provided outside hospital. The survey shows that the possibilities of effective social action in this sphere are limited. Loving daughters cannot be created by legislation, and many in this group had either no daughter or no love. Nor did it seem likely that existing social services could be deployed in this group very much more effectively than they were being used. They were either rejected by patients as irrelevant to their needs, or were overstrained in situations for which they were not designed. If the problem of insufficient basic care is to be overcome without overwhelming the hospital service, new ways of looking at the needs of old people and their families are required. What form these might take will be discussed in Chapter 16.

10   The Bonds of Strain

Few people reach middle age without living through the experience of an aged parent's illness. When this is prolonged, and when it leads to physical and mental incapacity, the illness can dominate the lives of the sons and daughters, deprive them of the enjoyment of normal social intercourse, and fill their days with labour and their nights with anxiety. Many relatives bear their burden of care with love and without complaint, but others are exposed to conditions so arduous that the stoutest heart cracks, and the physical and mental health of the helper reaches the brink of breakdown.

The geriatrician who, in the course of his domiciliary visit at the patient's side, saw for himself at close quarters the gigantic burden of care that was borne could not avoid feeling compassion and concern for those who had laboured long to care for the aged invalid. Even in cases where little could be done medically for the patient, it was justifiable to admit him to hospital primarily to relieve the strain on the relatives. Often, indeed, the plea was heard from the harassed daughter, 'Doctor, if you don't take my father into hospital, you will need to take me.'

In the study of 280 patients accepted for admission to the geriatric unit the research team assessed that the helpers of 141 patients were labouring under 'undue strain', defined as 'a state of exhaustion in the helper, occasioned by the patient's illness, which threatened the helper's own physical or mental well-being'. In eighty-nine of these cases relief of undue strain on relatives was cited as the main reason for admission of the patient to the geriatric unit. These cases will be analysed and described in the present and succeeding chapters.

Some indication of what it must be like to live with and care for an ill old woman emerges from the following letter from the son-in-law of a patient whose name had earlier been put on the waiting list for admission to the geriatric unit:

30, Kirkoswald Street,
Glasgow, E.2.
2nd May, 1967

Dear Sir/Madam,

With reference to my wife's mother, Mrs. Sarah Green, who resides with us at the above address, I should like to furnish you with some facts about Mrs. Green to let you realise my cause for writing. Mrs. Green has been with us over the past 12 years, due to her inability to look after herself, as she is now in her late seventies. Since June of last year her condition has meant constant attention to her by my wife and self. Twice she has fallen on the staircase necessitating a trip to the Royal Infirmary to have wounds stitched. Mr. Isaacs of the Geriatric Unit has visited her on two occasions since last June and shortly after his last visit in January a social worker called and advised us that Mrs. Green would be placed high on the priority list for admission. The aforementioned told us to contact Duke Street if conditions worsened. I am sorry that circumstances now force me to write, not asking but pleading for your help as my wife is reaching a stage now where I would not be surprised if she had a nervous breakdown.

Believe me this is no figment of my imagination as the work involved is tremendous. Her normal day means getting her mother up every morning at 6 a.m., dressing and washing her, help her downstairs to the living room. Her bed has to be stripped and changed every morning as it is saturated with urine, this entails a washing every day to keep a constant supply of clean bedding. Now we have started using incontinence pads to try and ease the burden. We also have to place them below her on the chair where she sits most of the day and I won't bother you with details of cushions, skirts etc. which are constantly needing changed as the stench is a source of embarrassment to anyone coming into our home. She is unable to go upstairs to the bathroom without help and as she is quite a heavy person, my wife is finding it more difficult each day to help her upstairs. We give her two sleeping tablets every night but she keeps calling out for my wife every morning at approximately 1 a.m. and thereafter almost continually until we get her up at 6 a.m. She then sits and dozes most of the day, sometimes coming away with unintelligent talk about dogs running about or someone's chasing her. Much of this we just accept but now we are forced to live a life with no social side at all as one of us has to stay in to let the other out for a few hours. My married daughter used to take a night to let us out but as she is expecting a baby in June quite logically she can

51

no longer come over from King's Park to do so. My wife has only one sister who is in Australia and all other relatives of Mrs. Green are deceased.

I have endeavoured to get the position of the circumstances over to you by means of writing and I am more worried about my wife's health than anyone else's.

I think after doing our duty for such a long period we are surely due a respite from it and be able to live our own life a little bit easier. It is to you therefore, that I earnestly ask if something can be done very soon for Mrs. Green, as I have tried to explain it is becoming more difficult every day to attend her, keeping her clean, and making her comfortable. For your consideration of this case my wife and I are sincerely grateful.

I remain, Yours sincerely,

Mr. A. McNee

The features of this case which are characteristic of those where 'undue strain' was recorded are: the long duration of Mrs Green's illness; her immobility, falls, incontinence and mental abnormality; the fact that her daughter was the only available helper; the burden of physical work by day and the disturbance of sleep by night; the lack of social life; and the impoverishment of the daughter's own marriage.

In determining whether in any given case strain should be classed as 'undue', the doctor and the social workers applied consistent standards. 'Strain' was defined as a state of physical and mental exhaustion of the helper, and was not a measure of the burdensomeness of the situation. A burden of care which was beyond the capacity of one helper might be borne with less difficulty by another. Some degree of strain is inherent in any situation where an ill old person has to be looked after at home. A helper's complaint of being tired or being tied to the house was not enough. The doctor and the social worker had to be convinced that there was a genuine threat of breakdown in the helper, and that this was wholly or largely attributable to the needs arising from the patient's illness, before a case was classified as one of 'undue strain'. It was only exceptionally that any real difficulty was encountered in the classification. All too often the strain under which the relative laboured was patently obvious in the lined face, her shadowed eyes, her twisting fingers, her sense of guilt and inadequacy at the cracking of her resolve to keep the patient at home as long as possible.

What factors were responsible for the undue strain suffered by so many of the relatives of these geriatric patients? As a first step to answering this question, the 141 patients whose relatives suffered undue strain were compared, in respect of a number of social and medical factors, with the forty-eight patients who received adequate care at home without undue strain. This comparison excluded the ninety-one patients already discussed who received insufficient basic care, although many of their relatives also experienced very severe strain. The detailed results are given in Part II, Tables 23 and 33 (pp. 140-1 and 145-6).

The important social factors distinguishing the 'strain' and 'no strain' groups proved to be the patient's age, marital status and household structure. Two groups of patients were most likely to cause strain—those aged eighty-five and over who were being looked after either by a very elderly spouse or by a 'child', herself an old-age pensioner, and those under the age of sixty-five whose daughters had young families of their own. Patients who lived alone caused less strain than did those who lived with a spouse or family, either because they were admitted to hospital at a relatively early stage of their illness or because relatives were able to get away from them for part of the day and to have an undisturbed night's sleep. The better-housed patients, and those from the higher social classes, seemed to cause more strain than the others, but this was probably because many poorly housed people of low social class lived alone and were admitted to hospital relatively early, whereas more of the well-housed lived with a son or daughter and remained longer at home.

This last explanation is supported by the comparison of the medical conditions of the two groups of patients. The patients who caused strain were much more ill and dependent, and had been so for much longer, than those where undue strain was absent. Nearly one-half of the strain cases were incontinent, more than half were mentally abnormal, and three-quarters were confined to bed or chair. One-third had been in a state of dependency for more than one year at the time of their referral, and another third had been dependent for between one month and one year. One-third of these patients died within three months of their admission to hospital.

The sources of help used by the two groups of patients are tabulated also in Tables 23 and 24 (pp. 140 and 141). In the strain cases the principal helper was most often an aged spouse or a middle-aged daughter, with the exception of the small group of comparatively young patients who were looked after by young married or unmarried children. Only about 15 per cent of the strain cases used the home help service, only 30 per cent had a district nurse, and the other domiciliary services were very seldom used.

These findings convinced us that in the eastern part of Glasgow in 1967 the dominant behaviour pattern was that those ill old people who had family members capable of caring for them were looked after at home. This was done predominantly by relatives, who sought little aid from hospitals or from domiciliary services. The family continued to care for the patient as the illness advanced throughout a long period of dependency, until a stage was reached where the severity and multiplicity of the patient's symptoms were so great that the burden of care overwhelmed the helpers. Then and only then did they seek the patient's hospitalization. Admission to hospital was at this stage unavoidable, otherwise the relatives would themselves have broken down. However, in many cases the disease had passed beyond the possibility of effective cure, the patient was approaching the end, and death took place within a short time of admission.

Many further questions arise from these findings. What factors were responsible for the strain on the relatives? Why was there reluctance to use the available services? What might be done to alleviate the strain? To answer these questions, we shall need to look more closely at the cases of strain.

11   The Sources of Strain

In the case of Mrs Green, described by her son-in-law's letter in the previous chapter, many strands intertwined to form the ropes of strain in which patient, daughter and family were bound. A multiplicity of causes was characteristic of the other cases of strain, but it was possible to classify these causes into three groups: factors in the patient, factors in the helper and factors in the helper's life-space. Although strain can only be fully understood through the interaction of these causes, it is convenient to consider the various factors separately.

Factors in the patient which caused strain were further divided into:

Physical disease   Personality
Mental disease   Environment

The following case illustrates the strain caused by physical incapacity. Mrs Colvin, a childless widow of seventy-five, had suffered from rheumatoid arthritis for ten years, but had remained semi-ambulant until six weeks before referral, when she took to bed with pyelonephritis. Her arthritis flared up and her joints became so exquisitely painful that she dreaded being moved, and could tolerate being lifted only all in one piece. She had urgency of micturition and required the commode frequently. The patient lived with an unmarried sister aged seventy-three, who had herself been in hospital one year previously with a myocardial infarction. During the day the sister obtained assistance from a home help and a neighbour, but she was alone with the patient all night. 'How I dread the nights,' she told the social worker. 'I go to bed so exhausted that I feel I could sleep for a month; but I dare not let myself fall over because I know that she will call, so I fight to stay awake waiting for her.'

The demands made as a result of physical incapacity were very heavy, involving lifting and laying of overweight helpless patients in far from ideal circumstances, day after day, night after night, without a rest or break for the worn-out helper. Often the physical strength required to sit a heavy helpless or resistive patient up in bed was very considerable—many of these patients, once they were in hospital, needed two or three nurses for this task—and it was almost beyond imagining how a frail elderly spouse could possibly have coped with such a situation. Yet somehow they managed, and indeed the physical burden seldom stood high in the complaints made by relatives who were under strain.

The bedfast patient was less of a strain than the unsteady ambulant one who was in danger of falling. The fear of a fall occurring was a potent cause of strain in the helper, as was the effort required to raise the fallen patient from the floor. An example was Mr Alexander, a widower of eighty-three, suffering from cerebral arteriosclerosis, who lived with his daughter, her husband and five children. His daughter had looked after him since his first fall a few months previously. The son-in-law was on permanent night shift, and the daughter was left in the house during the night with the old man and the children. Almost every night the patient rose to go to the toilet. 'I lie awake all night,' said the daughter, 'waiting for the thud. Sometimes I can manage with a struggle to get him up, sometimes I can't budge him and I just have to cover him with a blanket till my husband comes home from his work. We have a bottle and a commode—but see my father, you can't tell him anything. He won't listen to you.'

Loss of sleep due to the patient's demands for attention during the night was complained of by many relatives, particularly those who had a job to do during the day. Some patients required toileting up to half a dozen times a night, 'and if you don't run as soon as he calls', said one worn-out wife, 'he just does it in the bed, and then it's twice the work'. Others asked repeatedly for drinks or to have their pillows adjusted. Others insisted on getting up to the toilet themselves, despite warnings, and fell when they did so. This caused relatives to lie awake in the hope of forestalling a fall. One daughter knew she could not lift the patient, but was most reluctant to call a neighbour who had been most helpful in the past, as she had her own work to go to. 'The days aren't so bad,' said one wife, 'but if you don't get your night's sleep you're good for nothing the next day.'

In sixty-one patients one of the physical factors associated with strain was incontinence of urine or faeces, or both, a symptom which degraded the patient and reduced the helpers to a state of loathsome and endless drudgery. The round of stripping, changing, washing and laundering seemed unending, and the work was repellent and fatiguing. The subject of incontinence will be dealt with in detail in

Chapter 14.

Many other physical symptoms in patients were associated with strain in relatives. Patients with heart failure who were subject to attacks of breathlessness, especially during the night, were responsible for much anxiety and sleep loss. Those who were in pain and who requested frequent changes of position formed another group. Particularly exhausting were the younger patients with disabling diseases of very long standing, for example rheumatoid arthritis or multiple sclerosis, where the lengthy duration of the illness caused chronic exhaustion of the helper.

Great as was the strain caused by physical symptoms, that caused by mental abnormality was immeasurably greater. Time and again relatives told us, 'I don't mind the work, although at times I am worn out by it. It's the constant worry and anxiety, the fear that I will never know what she might do next.' The type of mental abnormality most often present in our patients and causing most strain was dementia. The following is a verbatim transcript of the description, given by the granddaughter of a demented old lady, of what her life with the patient was like.

'She brought me up, you know. She used to live with my uncle —her son—a man about forty-five and not in the best of health himself. His wife goes out to the Bingo two or three nights a week. There always has to be someone to stay in with the old lady. He didn't mind at first. She doesn't want you to sit and watch TV. She doesn't want to talk to you really. She just wants to sit and ask you about her mother and her father, her brothers and her sister. Well, it's all right maybe once or twice, but when it goes on and on it gets monotonous.

'She asks you to lift the window for her but she really just wants attention because she can do that herself. My uncle couldn't take it any more. She turns to hate you when she stays with you—well not really hate, you annoy her more than she annoys you. She is never content, can't sit at peace. She doesn't like to see you sitting. You must be up running around after her.

'There was a house going next door to me, and my uncle and aunt thought she would maybe be better on her own and asked me to get it for her. So I got her the house and we moved her into it. She likes it. I said I would cook for her and give her her meals. She lies late in the day. I get her up and help her to wash and dress. I sit her in her chair by the window. During the day she's all right when she can see people from the window. As night comes she gets fear into her. She sees someone in the street below and thinks maybe she knows them so she shouts at them to come up. It's embarrassing. She asks everybody about her mother and father. On and on and on until you feel like screaming at her, and she feels like screaming at you too.

'Sometimes her mind comes back and she says it's a terrible thing being like that. She says she has no pain but everything seems to be swimming. She says she can't think straight or positive. She just swims around and can't stop herself. Then I feel sorry for her. Other times I could strangle her. That's the way things are.

'I was always a happy person, but I saw my grandmother going like this and now I really don't feel I've got anything to live for. It builds up in you year after year. It really breaks you up to see her every day getting worse. You think of all the cruel things you say to her and you lie at night and ask God to forgive you. I was happy when she was in hospital. I felt marvellous because she was away from me. I could go up and see her but then I could leave her and forget her for a little.

'I don't think I could face the possibility of looking after her at home. I think I would be the first to die—I really would. I can't see any human being putting up with the awful strain. If it was my job to look after old people, that would be different because at the end of the day I could leave them and go home. But day in and day out I couldn't move but I'd be needed. When I go out for messages, in a shop I feel myself all going funny and I have to get home to see that everything is all right. My mother was the same. She used to look after my grandmother. When you are in the house you want to get out, but when you're out you can't wait to get back in. You're all mixed up inside. It's not the physical work of caring for her that's the real problem. If you're healthy enough you can cope with anything physical, but the mental strain is the worst. It's impossible. My aunt did her best to play fair but she has her own life to lead too.

'I have one daughter of six. She always loved her Great Granny but she's getting to be cheeky and really doesn't care about her any more. It's not nice to say such a thing about an old person but she torments the child all the time. She doesn't want her to go out to play and keeps telling her to come in. She tells her not to do this and not to do that. She even steals her sweeties off her. The child is getting to resent her more and more. Maybe it's because I don't have so much time for her now and she doesn't like it.

'People say it's terrible she has no one else to look after her and what's to happen to her. When you're with her you realize that you couldn't ask anybody to put up with it. What can we do?'

Mental abnormality, usually in the form of dementia, was present in seventy-nine of the patients whose care at home was associated with unbearable strain in the relatives. The symptoms of the disease adequately account for the strain which it engendered. Commencing insidiously with impairment of memory the disease slowly and relentlessly progresses, until its victims lose all comprehension of their surroundings and all the patterns of mature behaviour which they have acquired to enable them to live safely and sociably. As the disease advances abnormal patterns of behaviour escape from the repression usually imposed upon them, and the conduct of the victim becomes reprehensible. The manifestations of the disease are as varied as the personalities of the sufferers, but certain symptom patterns are commonly encountered. Loss of short-term memory was a potent cause of domestic accidents—the patient would put a kettle on the gas and forget to light it, or, having lit it, he would forget to take it off again, so that the vessel burned out. Loss of comprehension led to lack of self-criticism and of a sense of responsibility for actions. The mind became 'one-track' and the patient was able to think only of immediate gratification of his wishes without regard to consequences. Examples of the type of behaviour to which these abnormalities lead included: giving away money on impulse to strangers and later accusing others of having stolen it; dropping lighted matches on the carpet; losing money, pension books, spectacles, etc.; wandering from the house and getting lost; making extravagant and unnecessary purchases; returning to work at a place of former employment; dressing carelessly or inappropriately, perhaps leaving fly buttons open; going to bed with clothes on; refusing to wash.

In severe cases the patients became disorientated for time, place and persons. Many failed to recognize their closest relatives. This state of mind might simply be one of quiet bewilderment, but more often a delusional belief replaced the correct orientation. This was sometimes merely pathetic, as in the case of patients who called their own daughters 'Mother'. In other cases the dement projected quite unjustified feelings of hostility against a devoted daughter, who was addressed as 'nurse' or even as 'gaoler'. Disorientation for place prompted the belief in some patients that they were being held captive against their will in someone else's house, and they frequently wandered away in a vain search for their own house. Disorientation for time was responsible for the belief of some patients that the middle of the night was the time to rise and go out to work. Sleep reversal was another common behaviour pattern. The patient sat about drowsily all day and even refused to rise from bed, but at night he prowled restlessly around the house, sometimes all night long.

In the most severely demented patients regressive and atavistic behaviour patterns emerged. Excessive eating was common, and so too was food refusal (the latter sometimes in the belief that it was poisoned). Incontinence occurred often, as also did abnormal excretory behaviour patterns which were not true incontinence. These included soiling the lavatory floor; micturating against the bedroom wall, on the kitchen floor, or into a hat; handling and smearing faeces; parcelling up faeces in soiled underwear and concealing this in drawers and cupboards. Exposure and sexual advances were also encountered in this group.

The reaction which the abnormal thought, speech and behaviour of the dement aroused depended to some extent, especially in the early stages, on the insight and understanding of the relatives. It was difficult for some to appreciate that this old man, who refused to wash or who accused them of pocketing the pension money, had an organic illness, as surely as if his ankles had been swelling as a result of heart disease. So accusations led to recriminations, tension was generated and the bonds of strain began to tighten. The distress of other relatives was caused by feelings of shame at the patient's behaviour, and irrational guilt at the discovery that they now hated a parent whom they once had loved. A more general feeling was fear—fear that the house would be burned down, that the patient would gas himself or be killed in a street accident—'and then', one daughter said, 'I would never forgive myself.'

Strain on relatives was least in the case of patients living alone whose family were spared constant exposure to the abnormal personality, but anxiety was patent in this group, too. As one woman said of her demented mother who still lived alone, 'She is never out of my mind for one minute. Every time I go to her house I dread what I may find.' Here are a few further illustrative examples.

A husband living with his demented wife found that his life-long companion was a companion no longer. 'She sits all day muttering to herself, folding and unfolding a dish cloth, looking at me, not knowing who I am.'

The fifty-two-year old unmarried daughter of another demented old woman said, 'The minute I come here for my visit there she is waiting for me. She talks and talks and talks, but it is just a stream of rubbish. She won't let me do anything—read or knit or watch the television. And at 8 o'clock I've got to go to bed.' The complaint of another patient's married daughter was, 'She has got the idea that I am her mother. She calls me "Mother" and she follows me around all day holding on to me. It doesn't matter where I go or what I do, she is there like a shadow. She won't even let me go to the bathroom. But there's no conversation and she and I used to be such good pals. Sometimes I could weep, but most of the time I feel more like screaming.'

When Mrs Black became too forgetful to live alone she was

brought to her son's attractive home and given a room to share with his ten-year old son. The boy was terrified of her. She interfered with his homework and accused him of theft. The boy's school work suffered at a time when he was being prepared for entrance to a fee-paying school. The daughter-in-law resented the situation. 'My husband says the children have to learn to have compassion. That's all very well, but I can't stand by and watch my own son's happiness and future being sacrificed.'

Mrs Fotheringham had lived with her daughter and had shared a room with her granddaughter for many years. Her dementia developed insidiously, and when the granddaughter first complained about her, she was thought to be exaggerating. She had said that Mrs Fotheringham muttered and groaned all night long, got up, and just stood beside her bed staring at her. Then one day the granddaughter, now aged seventeen, packed her case and walked out. She went to stay with her boyfriend, and sent a message to her mother that she would not return home until Mrs Fotheringham was out of the house. The daughter was distraught. The girl was headstrong, determined, and meant what she said. The neighbours were talking. But how could she 'put her mother away'? She at length agreed to the compromise that Mrs Fotheringham would be admitted 'temporarily' to the geriatric unit for investigation, and the granddaughter returned home. The patient's 'temporary' admission duly became permanent.

Other forms of psychiatric disease, such as depressive illness, were less potent causes of strain than was dementia. But a factor in the patient which caused strain of extraordinary intensity and which was not in itself a disease was the personality of the patient. This cause of strain was manifest in those patients who had always been selfish, ill-tempered, demanding, autocratic and inflexible, giving little love and receiving little in return. When ill health deprived them of full participation in life they became even more selfish, irritable and demanding, so that, in the words of the relatives, 'there's no living with him'. Such services as were performed for patients of this type were given out of a cold sense of duty, and were received without gratitude or appreciation. One felt in the helper merely a sullen resentment. This pattern was found in two cases where one partner of a loveless marriage developed a chronic illness. The other, who had been almost on the point of separation, was obliged instead to perform menial bodily tasks for the patient. In a third case a domineering widower who had imposed puritanical sanctions on his thirty-seven-year old daughter and thwarted her hopes of matrimony continued to rule her life from his sick-bed, while she dutifully ministered to him and despised him in her heart. In a few other cases in this group the patient had a cold puritanical personality, and it may be more than a coincidence that the narrow religious teaching in these households had reinforced the domineering personality of the parent and had implanted guilt feelings in the children.

Factors in the patient's environment which were conducive to strain proved to be of very much less significance. Indeed, the statistical study showed that the worst-housed patients generated the least strain; while this seemed to be due not to living in a bad house but to the fact that more people in poor houses lived alone, the finding did conform with the experience of the doctor and the social worker. Relatives very seldom cited the patient's physical environment as an important factor in strain—apart from the distance which separated them from the patient's house. The factors which made the burden of caring for an ill old person overwhelming were, above all, the personality of the patient, the distortion of personality and behaviour caused by mental illness, and to a lesser extent the physical burden of providing night-and-day nursing care for the helpless.

12   The Victims of Strain

The group of people on whom fell the strain of caring for these aged patients were their husbands, wives and daughters, and to a lesser extent their sons, sons-in-law, daughters-in-law, sisters, nieces and grandchildren. In four cases it was a neighbour or friend who had been shouldering the whole burden and who could carry on no longer. All the patients in this group were very well cared for: they were fed, kept warm and clean, and given devoted nursing attention within the ability of the helper. Apart from the factors in the patient described in the previous chapter, it was possible to identify the following causes of strain in the helper and in the helper's life-space, that is the necessary activities which competed for the helper's time:

Age	Care of young children
Physical health	Employment
Mental health	Housing
Personality	Own marriage
Care of other dependent	Social activities

The ages of 'principal helpers' in cases of strain are recorded in Table 24 (p. 141). Of the twenty-five helpers who were themselves over the age of seventy, three-quarters were the wife or husband of the patient; most of the rest were sisters. They had carried on with their onerous task incredibly for weeks or months before appealing for help.

One household visited consisted of an eighty-nine-year old man with a history of frequent falls who was looked after by his eighty-eight-year old wife. She had on several occasions had to lift him off the floor when he fell. The husband was admitted to hospital where he improved so markedly that it was possible to send him home again. Three months later the doctor was called to the house again to find that this time it was the wife who had taken a stroke and the husband who was caring for her.

The mutual attachment of these long-married couples, and their amused tolerance of one another's foibles, removed many causes of strain, but the physical burden eventually proved too much for their great hearts. Second marriages were not always so happy, and the severe strain noted in some of these cases was due only in part to the age of the spouse, in part to a feeling almost of exasperation that an arrangement entered into late in life for mutual comfort should have led instead to an exhausting demand for care.

In widows and widowers of advanced old age the 'child' might herself feel too old for the task. In one household, the patient, his daughter and his two sons, who all lived with him, were all old-age pensioners. The average age of sons or daughters who were principal helpers was about fifty, but many were over sixty. At ages like this, helpers were not physically fit to carry the burden of care, and many suffered from diseases which made physical effort and sleep-loss most undesirable for them. The aged couple already described had one son only. He was sixty-one years old and had just come out of hospital after a myocardial infarction. His wife of fifty-eight was a diabetic, taking insulin. Once before when she had over-exerted herself she had gone into a coma, and she had been warned against doing anything similar again. Another old lady with rheumatoid arthritis was lifted and laid by a sister who was on the brink of cardiac failure, while the nursing of an elderly dement was in the hands of a forty-eight-year old daughter who had just completed a course of radiotherapy for cancer of the breast. Another dement, already referred to, was cared for by a schizophrenic son, temporarily discharged from a mental hospital.

In other cases the ill health of the helper was less clearly defined. Back strain, exhaustion and menopausal symptoms were often cited by the helpers as being among the reasons which contributed to the strain. Our impression was that few of these relatives were malingering or exaggerating.

A further group of relatives complained of physical symptoms, but were thought by the geriatrician to be suffering from psychiatric disturbances. They complained of headache, choking sensations or difficulty in swallowing, and when closely questioned it emerged that they had experienced similar symptoms at times of stress in the past. Another group were simply incapable of coping with the situation. These included a number of husbands and unmarried sons with no concept of domesticity, who were overwhelmed by the double task of caring for a disabled patient and running a house, did their best with such additional help as could be mustered, but were driven almost to frenzy by the unsolved problems of each day. We also identified a small number of inadequate people whose life history

64

revealed a pattern of failure to deal with stress, and who were submerged by the needs of the elderly patient. It would, we feel, be facile and wrong to dismiss these groups as 'reluctant helpers'. Their capacity to help was constitutionally small; their reaction to overload was to sit down and cry.

A subtle cause of strain in quite a few cases seemed to be the inability of a daughter or daughter-in-law to adopt a quasi-parental role towards the patient. They could not impose their will on the patient, as they might have been able to do with a stranger. This was particularly noticeable with patients who failed to wash or who had dirty excretory habits.

The ability of a helper to cope with the burden of care seemed to be related to her life experience. Those who had lived in the tenements of Glasgow's East End throughout the Hungry Thirties and the Second World War were inured to privation, and were no strangers to heavy unremitting physical work. Those who held a deep religious faith drew comfort from it, and expressed joy that they were given the opportunity to be of service. To those who lacked such a background the strain was harder to bear.

We come now to a group of factors causing strain which had in common that the demands made upon the relative to care for the patient encroached upon a fully occupied 'life-space'. This compelled the helper to discard from her life some activity which she valued, loss of which had implications for her and her own family.

Some people had a vacant life-space, and the care of an ill old person did not create strain, but was even welcomed as a life-space filler. This was the case with a childless widow of sixty-seven who looked after her seventy-five-year old neighbour in a block of pensioners' flats for many months without complaint, despite the fact that the patient weighed 15 stones, was bedfast and frequently incontinent. At the opposite pole was a sixty-six-year old widow who had a stroke and who was looked after by a thirty-year old married daughter with five children. Somehow the daughter had managed to go out to work, but when the patient took ill she abandoned her job, with a chain of disastrous consequences. Payments on furniture obtained on hire purchase were suspended, the family's holiday plans were abandoned, and the daughter's husband began to resent her frequent absences from the home and complained that he did not get his meals and that the children were neglected. Arguments flared up as each partner accused the other of selfishness, and, by the time the doctor was called, the daughter's marriage had been irreparably damaged.

This case illustrates the finding mentioned in Chapter 10 that strain was frequent amongst younger patients whose daughters were still involved in raising children, establishing themselves economically, and developing their own marriages. It is perhaps at this age that the life-space is most crowded, and that the many hours of work each day that the care of an ill old person at home demands are most difficult to find. In 'strain' cases, as in the cases of 'pre-occupation' described in Chapter 7, competing demands on the time of the helper included the care of young children and of other sick or dependent relatives.

The competing claim of employment is a more controversial matter. There are those who believe that some ill old people who could be cared for at home are instead sent into hospital because their relatives prefer to go out to work. It has been suggested that in such cases it might be appropriate to pay a daughter to stay at home and care for the patient, and indeed such schemes are in operation in a number of places. Amongst the geriatric patients in the present survey whose daughters were in employment, the majority were widowed, divorced or unmarried. They were the sole wage-earners, and dreaded the loss of their jobs if they stayed off work.

Then there was a small group of self-employed people with little businesses of their own—a dairy, newsagent's or confectioner's—who could not afford to hire labour or to close the shop. Another small group included professional people with a high sense of vocation (for example schoolteachers) or women holding positions of responsibility (for example a private secretary to the managing director of a firm) who had special cause to find difficulty in abandoning their work. Next, there was a small group of daughters who cared all day for a demanding patient, and who felt they simply had to take a part-time job in the evenings to get out of the house in order to keep themselves from going insane. There was thus very little scope for the type of help referred to. Thirty-one relatives of geriatric patients in the present series gave up or stayed off work in order to care for the patient, for periods varying from one week to three years. All who stayed off temporarily went to their own doctors and had themselves 'put on the panel'—a practice in which the general practitioners seemed perfectly happy to collude—and were thus able to draw sickness benefit.

One patient whose daughter found great difficulty in staying off work was Mrs Stapleton. An obese, deaf lady of eighty, she had severe osteo-arthritis of the hips and knees, and required to be lifted bodily out of bed and on to a chair. She lived with her fifty-six-year old daughter, the daughter's husband who had retired after a coronary thrombosis, and one of their daughters, a medical student. Their other daughter, a nurse, was married and lived nearby, but had a young baby. The daughter, the sole wage-earner of the household, was the millinery buyer for a department store. Her duties included monthly buying visits to London, attending company

66

meetings and being entertained by manufacturers. She rose every morning at six, and before she left for work at 8.30 she did the housework, prepared the day's meals, got the patient up, toileted her, and dressed and fed her. On her return at night she served a meal, completed the housework and put the patient back to bed. On some days Mrs Stapleton was too ill to be left. These relapses had a habit of coinciding with her daughter's trips to London. Then emergency plans had to be brought into action. The student granddaughter stayed off classes, the nurse granddaughter brought her baby, and with the help of the anginal son-in-law they managed. But the patient screamed and said no one could lift her except her daughter. The latter dreaded staying off work in case she was dismissed—'and then where would I be at my age?' she asked. Mrs Stapleton was admitted to hospital to relieve the strain on the family, but it was later decided to keep her in permanently.

The employment of married women is an established part of modern living. The economy of the country depends on it, and so too does the economy of many a family. The employment of married women also offers them an opportunity of widening their roles and increasing their social contacts. This enlargement of the social and economic role of the married woman inevitably obstructs her role as mother, wife and daughter. The choice which she faces when a parent becomes disabled and requires her help is not simply one of personal preference, but has implications on her own life and on that of her family. Faced with this choice a substantial number of women in the present series gave up their work, but in so doing they unavoidably set up currents of strain.

There were perhaps half a dozen cases in the present series, certainly not more, where it might have been thought reasonable to pay a daughter to give up her work in order to look after the patient. On completion of active hospital treatment a proportion of patients could perhaps be sent home rather than cared for in a long-stay unit, if a daughter could be financially compensated for giving up her job to look after the patient. We have no figures for this group, but believe the number, in our area at any rate, to be very small.

We turn now to another source of strain—a change in living arrangements necessitated by the patient's illness, when either the patient was taken to live with a family member, as happened in nineteen cases, or when someone else (usually a daughter) moved in to live with the patient, as happened in thirteen cases. This was least stressful when the house was large enough for the patient to be given a room of his own. This was rarely the case in the present survey, and a move of this type generally involved loss of privacy and overcrowding, with all the attendant arguments, conflicts and discontent. One source of strain in this situation was the disturbance of the conjugal life of the patient's daughter and son-in-law. Usually they moved out of their own bedroom to give it to the patient, and slept on a convertible settee in the living room, where they were subject to disturbance by late home-coming teenagers. Or the patient was given the room of a child who then came to sleep with the daughter and son-in-law. In one case a family with six children living in a house with one room and a kitchen took the wife's bedfast old mother to stay with them and gave her a room to herself, while the rest of the family somehow found somewhere to sleep. The experience of this survey suggested that a three-generation household requires a three-generation house. In its absence strain is very liable to occur. Social life and leisure were the first activities to be dislodged from the life-space of a relative caring for an ill old person. This was a sacrifice which most relatives willingly bore. Daughters would admit with a wan smile, when directly asked, that they had not been out alone with their husbands for months or years. However, there were more circumstances where loss of social life was a cause of severe strain.

An attractive unmarried girl of twenty-five had given up work three years previously to look after her mother who had become helpless as a result of multiple sclerosis. 'It wasn't so bad at first,' she said. 'My friends used to come round and sit with me, and occasionally my cousin or my married sister would let me out to go to the pictures or a dance. But gradually they stopped coming one by one, and my mother had a row with my cousin, so she stopped coming too. My mother doesn't like me to go out, and I suppose I have just got used to it. But at times I could scream.' This girl refused the offer of holiday admission for the patient. 'What would be the use?' she said, 'I've no one to go away with.'

A final factor which loomed large in many cases was the strain on a daughter's own marriage created by her need to look after her aged parent. This was influenced by the degree to which the old person had been absorbed into or had stood aloof from, the daughter's family. Here is a typical example. Mrs Crane was a formidable old lady who suffered from cardiac failure and could do little for herself. A bachelor son lived with her, and cared for her at night, while during the day she was nursed by a married daughter. Many years previously the daughter had mortally offended her by marrying a man of different religion, and Mrs Crane, by her acid comments on the situation and her subsequent attempts to interfere in the religious upbringing of her grandchildren, was persona non grata in the daughter's household. The daughter had long since forgiven these indiscretions, and would have greatly preferred nursing the patient in her own home to travelling daily by three buses in each direction to Mrs Crane's home. 'But,' she said, 'my husband won't have her in the house. He says, if she comes, he goes. And he's my husband ...

In families which were warm, close-knit and united, the illness of a parent evoked a co-operative response. Mrs Lewis had an exceptionally sweet and loving nature. When she became bedfast and incontinent her three married daughters worked out a rota whereby each took it in turn to spend twenty-four hours with her, nursing her, running her home and sitting up all night. The system lasted for three months, and the daughters' own families adjusted their ways of life uncomplainingly. Eventually the health of two of the daughters broke down, and the third turned to the geriatric unit for help.

This pattern was not usual. More often, when one daughter took on the care of the patient other members of the family guiltily disappeared from the scene, as in the following case. Mrs Wotherspoon suffered a stroke at the age of sixty-two and made a partial recovery. When she was ready to leave hospital the large family held a conference, and it was agreed that an application should be made to the Corporation Housing Department for a house to be allocated to one of the daughters, in exchange for Mrs Wotherspoon's former house. This was duly arranged and the patient came to live with the daughter. The other sons and daughters promptly ceased to visit. Over the next two years the daughter, who already had six children, suffered a threatened miscarriage, a full-term pregnancy, a post-partum haemorrhage and a hysterectomy. On each of these occasions a request was received for Mrs Wotherspoon's re-admission to the geriatric unit. The other sons and daughters produced tenuous excuses as to why they were unable to take the patient. One of them confessed his true reason to the social worker. 'The way I look at it is this,' he said. 'She got a house out of it, didn't she? Right! She took on the responsibility, didn't she? Well then, it's got nothing to do with me.' Cases of this nature were often traced back to old family feuds related to money. The strain of caring for the patient was made much worse by the daughter's resentment at the unequal distribution of the burden.

In case after case in this series the doctor and the social worker witnessed the exhaustion of the helper, or experienced something of the anguish and torment occasioned by the conflicting demands of caring for the patient and solving all the other problems of family and economic life. An astonishing and regrettable feature was the small amount of help that this overburdened group of patients drew from the domiciliary services. Only 1 in 3 used the assistance of a district nurse, only 1 in 4 had a home help, and the other statutory and voluntary services were very rarely used. This non-use of services was not due to non-availability. The services which were provided were not those which the relatives needed: the services which the relatives needed have not yet been properly identified. The majority of relatives knew of only one service which would be able to relieve them of their burden, and that was permanent admission to hospital. This was a solution which many were anxious to avoid. They had promised themselves to allow the old person the privilege of dying in his or her own bed, so they struggled on until they reached the limit of their strength, and then were overwhelmed with guilt at requesting hospitalization.

The problem of strain will not be easily solved. Domiciliary services that really meet needs are required, although it remains problematical whether such services would be used by those most in need. This problem is discussed further in Chapters 15 and 16. Perhaps the most effective change would be the education of doctors and families of old people to think of the geriatric unit as a place to be sought out, not one to be avoided, so that effective treatment can be given early whenever possible, and the burden of disability to be cared for in the community can be reduced to more manageable proportions.

No one could work with the relatives of the geriatric patients of Glasgow, as we did, without developing a profound admiration for their devotion and self-sacrifice, and their willing acceptance of a gigantic burden. No one could retain for a moment the absurd, oft-refuted, but still prevalent belief that people don't care what happens to old folk. But still one can ask whether the Health Service of a highly-taxed welfare state should have to depend so much on its unsung heroes and heroines, the middle-aged and elderly housewives.

13 The Triangles of Dependency

Geriatricians are often reminded that the view of the elderly which they obtain from a geriatric unit is distorted. It is quite wrong, one is told, to generalize about 'all old people' on the basis of experience with the small fraction of the aged who occupy geriatric hospital beds, ignoring the 95 per cent who live in their own homes. This seems a valid criticism. It has been taken seriously by a number of geriatricians who have made studies of old people in the community, and it seemed to us very desirable that our view of the problems of ill old people should be put into proper perspective by a community study of our own.

We chose death as the starting point of our study. We argued that, since more people are now living beyond the age of sixty-five, more people are dying after attaining the age of sixty-five. What happens, we wondered, to these people in the period immediately preceding their death? How many of them die in hospital, and how long do they remain in hospital before dying? In which type of hospital ward do they spend their last days? How many die at home, and what care do they receive there during their final illness? For how long are those who die in hospital ill at home before their last admission to hospital?

The method used for this community survey is described in detail in Part II. We obtained information about every person usually resident in the City of Glasgow who died during the year 1968 and who was aged sixty-five years or over when he died. There were 7,610 deaths. For all those who died in hospital we determined the type of hospital ward in which death took place, and the duration of stay in hospital immediately preceding death. We studied in more detail a sample of 250 of these 7,610 deaths by interviewing the bereaved relatives about the circumstances of the patient's illness at home which preceded his death at home or his final admission to hospital. Tables 36 to 56 (pp. 147 - 60) give full results of those enquiries.

The findings of this large-scale community survey gave no grounds for complacency, and no reason for believing that we had in any way exaggerated the plight of the aged. On the contrary, they provided additional evidence of the presence in the elderly of a vast reservoir of disease and disability. And even this understated the problem, since our enquiries were directed only towards the period which immediately preceded death, and took no account of illness at other stages of old age.

We first investigated the place of death. Just over one-third of the elderly Glaswegians whose deaths were registered in 1968 died in their own beds. The proportion who died at home was much the same for the two sexes and at all ages, but was higher for married people than for the single or the widowed. The proportion who died in hospital tended to fall with increasing age of the subject, particularly among women; this was due in part to the large number of very old ladies who died in private nursing homes or in residential homes. Among those who died in hospital, a striking change occurred with increasing age in the type of ward in which death took place. Most of those who were under the age of seventy-five at death died in 'acute' medical or surgical wards, and only comparatively few in geriatric or psychiatric wards. With increasing age at death this pattern was reversed: of those who were aged eighty-five years or over at death only a minority died in medical and surgical wards, the majority dying in geriatric and psychiatric wards.

Even more striking was the relationship between age, place of death and duration of final stay in hospital which preceded death. For those who died in hospital and who were aged between sixty-five and seventy-four when they died, the average duration of final hospital stay was 85 days; for those who were aged between seventy-five and eighty-four at death, it was 182 days. For men aged eighty-five and over the period of final hospital stay was 212 days, and for women in the same advanced age group it was no less than 399 days. The older a person was when he died the longer he spent in hospital in his final illness.

These figures for hospital stay were related to the ward in which death occurred. For patients aged sixty-five and over who died in a medical ward the average duration of final hospital stay was 31 days, and for those who died in a surgical ward it was 28 days. For men and women who died in a geriatric ward the average figures were 184 and 226 days respectively, while for those who died in a psychiatric ward the figures were 923 and 1,152 days. It is seen that prolonged survival of the very old in geriatric and especially in psychiatric wards was the reason for the very long duration of final hospital stay of those who died in advanced old age.

These figures can be expressed in the form of 'average hospital bed-days per death'. This average is obtained by dividing, for each age and sex group, the total number of days spent in hospital in final illness of those who died in hospital by the total number of deaths in that age-sex group, that is including in the denominator those who died at home as well as those who died in hospital. This calculation gave figures which ranged from 49 days for men aged from sixty-five to seventy-four to 181 days for women aged eighty-five and over. This means that on average every old woman who died in Glasgow in 1968 and who was aged eighty-five years or over when she died occupied a hospital bed for the last six months of her life.

The increase of 36 per cent of the population of Scotland aged seventy-five and over which is expected to take place between 1966 and 1986 will bring a disproportionately large demand for long-term hospital care in the period immediately preceding death, quite apart from the demand at other times in the old person's life.

The number of deaths of old people which occur in hospital depends on the number of hospital beds and other facilities, for example for domiciliary and residential care, which are provided. We therefore turned our attention to a study of the final illness of those old people who died at home, and to the home phase of care of those who subsequently entered hospital and died there. In this study, too, we found nothing which led us to believe that our concept of old people's needs had been in any way exaggerated.

In the sub-sample of 250 patients whose relatives were interviewed after their death, 116 had died at home. Of these, 1 in 6 had suffered from the inability to walk, incontinence or mental abnormality, or any combination of these symptoms, for one year or longer before death, and 1 in 3 had suffered from these symptoms for more than one month. The 134 patients who died in hospital had an even greater toll of disability. One-quarter of them had had one or more of these three symptoms of dependency for more than one year at home before final admission to hospital, and nearly one-half had had such symptoms for more than one month. These symptoms too were closely related to age at death. Taking together those who died at home and those who died in hospital, the proportions who were dependent at home for more than one year were 16 per cent for those aged from sixty-five to seventy-four, 22 per cent for those aged from seventy-five to eighty-four and 31 per cent for those aged eighty-five and over. The corresponding proportions who were dependent for more than one month were 37, 43 and 58 per cent respectively.

The small sample differed a little from the larger one in that more females than males died at home, while with increasing age of the subjects at death there was an increasing tendency for death to take place in hospital. This may have been because the East End of Glasgow, from which the smaller sample was drawn, lacked private nursing homes and residential homes. In their marital status and living arrangements the subjects who died at home differed little from those who died in hospital. For example, subjects who lived alone were represented almost as much among those who died at home as amongst those who died in hospital. The only substantial social difference detected between the groups was amongst those subjects who had no children in the locality. Many more of this group died in hospital than at home.

What medical factors influenced the place of death? This question was approached by comparing the presence and duration of the symptoms of dependency in the two groups of subjects. Immobility and incontinence occurred just as often—in fact slightly more often— amongst the subjects who died at home as they did in those who died in hospital, but 'mental abnormality' was present in only one-sixth of those who died at home, compared with two-fifths of those who entered hospital. Nearly one-third of all the subjects went through a period of mental abnormality at home, and three-quarters of these were subsequently admitted to hospital. Very long duration of a state of dependency also influenced the place of death. Subjects in whom dependency lasted for up to one year were no more liable to die in hospital than at home, but of those who were dependent for more than one year two-thirds entered hospital in their final illness; only one-third of them remained to die at home.

The burden of caring for these dying old people at home fell very largely on the elderly spouses and middle-aged daughters of the subjects, assisted by other relatives and kindly neighbours. The home help and district nursing services were of great value to those who used them, but this was a pathetically small proportion of those who could have benefited from them. A distressingly large number of old people died at home in inadequate circumstances, or in conditions which caused severe strain to their relatives.

This enquiry did not seek to determine all the reasons why some subjects died at home while others entered hospital, although it did demonstrate that subjects with no children in the neighbourhood, those with mental abnormality and those with a very prolonged state of dependency were especially prone to enter hospital in the course of their final illness. The study also revealed the enormous amount of disability which occurred during the final illness of old people, and how very much of this had to be dealt with in the subject's home, irrespective of whether death took place at home or in hospital.

The main conclusion of these community studies was that the grim picture of illness and disability in advanced old age which the geriatrician observes daily is not a distortion of the plight of old people in general. In fact, even the geriatrician sees only a fraction of the total burden. Death comes quickly and cleanly to but a few of those who survive into extreme old age. For many of them life lingers long after they lose the capacity for self-care, and their closing days are spent in a state of dependency on others. The longer they survive the longer on average does the state of dependency endure. When a combination of medical disability (especially mental infirmity) and social disadvantage eventually compels their entry into hospital they are still, on average, merely approaching the half-way mark in their long decline from independence to death.

These conclusions can be represented in the form of diagrams which display the 'triangles of dependency' (see Figure 5). The first diagram represents three streams of old people who died at home at the ages of sixty-five, seventy-five and eighty-five respectively. The older they were when they died the longer was the period of dependency which preceded death. The second diagram illustrates the finding that for those who died in hospital, the greater the age at death the longer was the period spent in hospital before death and the longer was the period of dependency at home preceding admission to hospital.

These results came from a random sample of the elderly population of Glasgow, and not from a selected group of geriatric patients. The graph in Figure 6 shows the growth in the population of Scotland aged sixty-five and over in the past twenty years, and the anticipated growth over the next twenty years. It serves as a reminder of the magnitude and urgency of the problem which the Survival of the Unfittest poses to us.

Finally, let us briefly consider, why do the unfit survive? Why do they survive unfit? The reason is because lethal disease is treatable and non-lethal disease is not. Many of the once-fatal maladies of the elderly, such as pneumonia and fractured neck of femur, are effectively cured by modern medicine, while the non-lethal diseases of the brain, the heart and circulation, the muscles and joints, the vision and hearing, exert their baneful effects unchecked, or only partially relieved. For some of these non-lethal but socially intensely disruptive diseases, most notably 'senile dementia', medicine has yet to find not merely a cure, not merely a means of prevention, but a basic understanding of its cause. For other diseases of the aged, such as atherosclerosis, some progress is being made towards developing methods of prevention, but it seems likely that these measures will have to be applied early in life if the effects of the disease on function in old age are to be avoided. In yet other diseases which cripple in late life, such as rheumatoid arthritis, effective methods of treatment are available, but they require early diagnosis

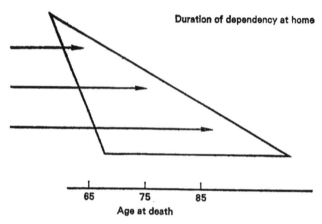

Figure 5 The triangles of dependency

    (a) For subjects who died at home, the greater the age at death the longer was the period of dependency preceding death

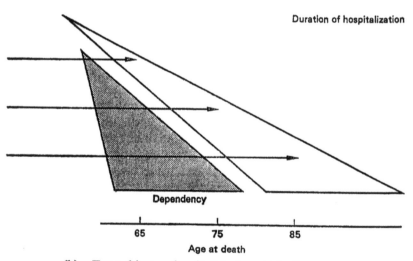

    (b) For subjects who died in hospital, the greater the age at death the longer was the period spent in hospital before death and the longer was the period of dependency at home preceding admission to hospital

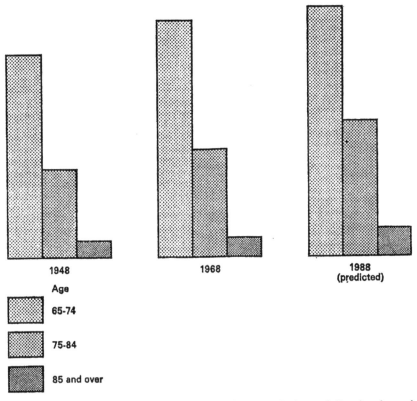

1948   1968   1988 (predicted)

Age

65-74

75-84

85 and over

Figure 6   Changes in the structure of the population of Scotland aged sixty-five and over from the Registrar General's reports and projection

and elaborate surgical treatment; the economic and administrative problems of bringing the right treatment to the right patient at the right time are so great that an effective solution seems equally remote. In a few other diseases of the very old impressive advances are being made, but ironically the greatest progress is in the ever-improving organization of medical and social services in late life, which promote the Survival of the Unfittest. Man's strength and intellect decline while his capacity to survive increases. Man has learned to outlive the vigour of his body and the wisdom of his brain, but he has not yet learned how to provide, from the society which he has created, for the new needs of those who survive unfit.

14 Incontinence

Throughout this book many references have been made to incontinence of urine or faeces. In the present chapter this information will be brought together and some new data added. This symptom is the ultimate degradation of old age, causing misery in the patient, a burden of labour to the relatives and a sense of despair to many in the medical and nursing professions. Moreover, it was the fear of wetting the bed which impelled many a frail old person to essay the journey from bed to bathroom by night, which ended for some in a catastrophic fall and a night-long exposure on the floor.

The wretched sufferer from incontinence proceeds from dread of his affliction, coupled with anxiety and shame, through increasingly vain efforts to control it, to an ultimate state of apathy and unawareness. Families display a range of emotions, from sympathy to intolerance. Some find it difficult to accept the involuntary nature of the condition, and unnecessarily aggravate the situation by adjurations to which the patient is unable to respond. The gates of sociability clang shut in the home of the incontinent patient. Friends absent themselves, and behind closed doors the unceasing work of washing and cleaning and mopping goes on, and the stale odours linger.

The following report of the case of a Mrs Twaddle may convey some impression of life among the incontinent. As the doctor entered the house, hardened to such scenes though he was, he was almost overwhelmed by the all-pervasive smell of urine and the billowing clouds of steam which emanated from the room. He was in the kitchen where a bed had been placed for the patient. The room resembled a Chinese laundry with rows of washing everywhere, and penetration into it was impeded by rows of wet sheets and napkins criss-crossing the room and flapping their damp folds into the doctor's face. The doctor had been called to advise on the management of a sixty-three-year old diabetic woman who had suffered a stroke eighteen months previously for which she had refused hospital treatment. She had remained in bed ever since, and for the past twelve months had been persistently incontinent of urine. Recently the skin of a wide area of her back and buttocks had become seriously excoriated by what proved to be a monilial infection. This had stimulated her to summon the family doctor, who in turn had called in the geriatric service. When Mrs Twaddle took her stroke she came to stay with her younger daughter. An older daughter lived far away and, preoccupied with the care of her own large family, was unable to be of much help. Two married sons in Glasgow were also only rare visitors, so the work fell on one pair of shoulders. This daughter, aged thirty, had six young children of her own, two of them still in nappies and only two at school.

The atmosphere in the house was tense. The proceedings were opened by the patient who delivered a spirited attack on the general practitioner: he was accused of negligence, impudence and lack of concern. The daughter then gave her account of the situation, demanding immediate action from the geriatrician. He meantime surveyed the room, noting the patches of condensed steam on the wall, the pools of water under the bed, the overhead pulley straining at its ropes, and the assortment of patched and threadbare sheets, pyjamas, nightdresses, napkins, cotsheets and drawsheets which hung from the pulley, lay over the ropes or were spread out over chairs, tables and any other article of furniture that served the purpose. The daughter was telling her tale. She rose at 7 a.m. to get her husband off to work and the children to school. The day was more than fully occupied with shopping, cooking, serving meals, housework and all the chores of a large family, but to this was added her mother's constant requests for attention and the almost ever-present need to change the bed. There was always so much to do that it was not until 11 p.m., when the family were all settled, that she was able to start the main washing, although she always tried to rinse linen as soon as it was fouled. The washing often went on till 3 or 4 in the morning. The daughter was able to keep going only because her husband worked on shifts, and sometimes he put the children out to school and let her sleep later in the morning.

In this case the patient was admitted to hospital, her diabetes was controlled, her skin healed, her output of urine was reduced, the degree of incontinence diminished, and a trial was made at rehabilitation. But she was so used to inactivity that treatment achieved only a limited success, and the small gain would have been lost if she had returned to the previous intolerable conditions. So Mrs Twaddle remained in hospital, where her diet was strict, her skin was kept clean and there was no need to live in a laundry. There she occupied a bed in a long-stay unit and was still alive one year later.

The high incidence of incontinence in old people is borne out by the finding that, among the 250 subjects drawn at random from the population who died after attaining the age of sixty-five, one-third had been incontinent at home at some time before their death. In this sample 1 person in every 7 was incontinent at home for more than one month, 1 in every 25 for more than one year, and 1 in every 80 for more than five years. Since some two-thirds of all deaths occur after the age of sixty-five, this means that (if this small local sample truly reflects the national incidence) nearly one-quarter of the population experience incontinence at home before their death; to these must be added the many who are incontinent only in hospital, those who are incontinent at an earlier stage of life, and the incontinent among those who die before the age of sixty-five.

The prevalence of incontinence in the community cannot be calculated from this data without making unjustifiable assumptions, but there may well be, at any one time, as many as 100,000 incontinent people in the United Kingdom—excluding the much larger number of women with stress incontinence.

There must be few other symptoms in the whole field of medicine which afflict so many sufferers, and which attract so little interest from the medical profession. With a few honourable exceptions the problems of incontinence, its causation and treatment, are ignored in our medical schools. One reason for this must be the erroneous impression of its incidence that medical students and doctors in teaching hospitals receive, since, in Glasgow at any rate in the past, the method of admission operated in a manner which tended to limit the number of elderly incontinent patients entering teaching hospitals. It will be recollected that only 8 per cent of patients aged sixty-five and over admitted to medical wards were incontinent on admission, compared with 51 per cent of those admitted to the geriatric unit.

Incontinence was equally common in the geriatric patients in the main series. Its incidence was not influenced by the marital or family status of the sufferer, or by his housing or social class. Incontinence was no more common in those patients over the age of seventy-five than in those between the ages of sixty-five and seventy-four. Nearly three-quarters of the patients who were incontinent when they applied for admission to the geriatric unit died within one year. These findings give support to a generally gloomy view of incontinence. In most old people the condition is caused by irreversible damage to the cerebral mechanism controlling bladder and bowel evacuation, and is accompanied by other manifestations of brain damage, notably disturbances of balance and intellectual impairment. But the better side must not be overlooked; 15 per cent of patients who were incontinent on admission to the geriatric unit went home within three months of admission and were fully continent at the time of their discharge. The condition is not always irreversible. There are cases where the incontinence represents an imbalance between the forces controlling the bladder and those depriving it of its control. It may be that the balance has been overturned by one small factor—concurrent illness, confinement to bed, fear or infection. Correction of this factor, aided by the adoption of a hopeful and helpful attitude by the nursing staff, can restore confidence, competence and continence. Modern nursing has at its disposal a number of techniques designed to aid this process and to reduce the burden.

However, the case of Mrs Twaddle shows how far removed is the practical management of incontinence in the patient's home from what could be achieved if modern methods were properly applied. Was Mrs Twaddle an exception? Or were there more like her? To find this out the last 100 patients in the geriatric series were surveyed. Amongst them were twenty patients who had been incontinent for two days or more before referral (see Table 35, pp. 146-7). These patients were being cared for at home by a spouse, a daughter or other relative, or in some cases where the patients lived alone, only by neighbours and home helps. Only 11 of the 20 were using incontinence pads, which are as elementary a necessity for incontinent patients in bed as are nappies for babies; but unlike nappies they are supplied free on the National Health Service. It is a dismal commentary on communication in the swampy field of incontinence that this basic item of equipment, which halves the Augean task of caring for the patient and which can be supplied at the stroke of a doctor's pen, was in so many cases lacking. Incontinence pads are by no means the sole answer to the problem, and they raise difficulties of their own. They are too small and not sufficiently absorbent, and the material often comes apart when very wet and adheres to the patient's skin. They are of value only to the bedfast, unless used in conjunction with plastic underpants, a solution used by none of the patients. And furthermore there are problems in their disposal. In seven of the eleven households they were burned acridly on an open coal fire. In the other four households, which were in a smokeless zone, the soiled pads were wrapped in newspaper and dropped surreptitiously after dark into the dustbin (which was emptied once a week). There were no dwellers in high flats in this group, but the problem of how to dispose of soiled pads in these vertiginous circumstances presented itself on other occasions, and was solved by the use of a common garbage chute.

Soiled linen had to be washed once, twice or more often each day. Only four of the twenty households had a washing machine, and only ten (including these four) had a running hot water supply. So in many homes the daily routine for the aged spouse of the incontinent patient was to heat kettles of water on the stove or

81

fire, wash the fouled linen in the single sink which served for all domestic and culinary purposes, and drape the soggy sheets over chairs and clothes horses in front of the fire. Six of the twenty households were more enterprising in the face of these laundering difficulties. One sent the fouled linen to a commercial laundry, and two washed it in a laundrette, though in none of these cases was the management made aware of the use to which their machinery was being put. The daughter of one patient and the home help of another wrapped each day's store of fouled linen in brown paper, and gingerly carried it through the streets to their own homes, where they washed it in their own washing machines. Finally, there was one daughter who lived too far away for this last expedient, so she brought a large suitcase with her each day, loaded it up with the urine-soaked sheets, and boarded the bus back home. She was acutely embarrassed by the bus conductor's witticisms on the lines of 'Going your holidays again, hen?', and by the subsequent strange glances as the pervasive odours escaped from the suitcase and wafted their way through the vehicle. But not one of these twenty patients was seen by a health visitor or was offered the services of the Local Authority laundries; not one received practical advice or help from the general practitioner on the use of appliances, drugs, bladder drill, adaptations to clothing or any other modern method of management; and not one received financial recompense for the cost of laundering, which was, in patients using commercial facilities, some £2 per week (at 1967 prices). However, 12 of the 20 did receive valuable help in stripping the bed and cleaning the patient from the district nurse, but the nurses came only once or twice a day, and the relatives (when there were relatives) or the home help (when there was a home help) were left to get on with it for most of the time. It is small wonder that hospital admission was looked upon as the only solution for these wretched patients.

The blame for this appalling state of affairs must rest squarely on the shoulders of the medical profession, no less affected than any other section of the populace by the repugnance which dripping urine and exuding faeces engender. Every medical student is taught minutely about leaking valves in the heart, but few ever hear mention of leaking bowels and bladders. It is primarily the doctor's task to draw attention to the human misery which this dismal symptom creates, to study its causes, to develop better methods of management and to ensure that existing knowledge, even at the elementary level of using incontinence pads, is widely disseminated and effectively applied. Local Authorities and other branches of the Health Service deserve their share of the blame for lack of imagination and insufficient commitment to the problem, but they have not been given the lead from the medical profession to which they might well have responded. Incontinence tells *in parvo* the whole tale of ill old people. More research and new methods are desperately needed, certainly, but how much unnecessary misery could be removed immediately if only existing knowledge was applied to the Mrs Twaddles of today.

15   Community Care

The expression 'community care' is applied to the services available outside hospital to people who need help, other than financial, to enable them to live a satisfactory life. Community care has to serve a wide variety of people, from the new-born infant to the valetudinarian. Our concern with community care in this study was not with the service as a whole, which we believe to have been an excellent one, but solely with its use by the ill old people referred to the geriatric unit. Specifically, we wanted to know to what extent community care was a substitute for hospital treatment. Briefly, our conclusions were that the services were of the utmost value to those who used them, but they reached only a fraction of those in need; even among these, too often the wrong people were receiving the wrong service at the wrong time.

Details of the utilization of the domiciliary services by the subjects in our surveys are given in Tables 27 to 30, 34, 55 and 56 (pp. 142-4, 146, 159 and 160).

The most important domiciliary service for the aged is the home help service, and in 1967 Glasgow was comparatively well off in this respect (see Table 3, p. 127). The city employed some two thousand home helps, and was able to provide a service to all qualifying applicants for between two and four hours a day, six days a week. In special cases help could also be given at weekends and in the evenings. Under very exceptional circumstances, full care up to eight hours per day could be provided for a very limited period only. Virtually any old person in need of help could obtain it for a period of eight weeks (for example after discharge from hospital) at a charge varying with household income. This charge ranged from 2s. (10p) per day for old people living alone to a maximum of nearly £2 per day. Thereafter continuing need was assessed, and in certain circumstances help was given for a reduced charge. In other cases, for example where the patient had a son or daughter living in the city, the rules required that a full charge was made, which was frequently greater than the family could afford to pay.

Only one-quarter of the geriatric patients in the main survey had a home help at the time of their referral for admission. Home helps were used by 1 in 5 of those patients who were aged sixty-five to seventy-four, 1 in 4 of those aged seventy-five to eight-four, and 1 in 2 of those aged eighty-five and over. The use of home helps was greatest for those living alone, next for old couples living together and least for old people living with a family. Men used home helps less than women did, but this was mainly because there were more very old women, and more living alone. Home helps were used most by patients whose disability was of moderate degree and intermediate duration.

It seemed that the presence of a home help to assist a disabled old person living alone delayed the patient's referral to the geriatric unit, but the patient needed so much more aid than the home help could give that eventually referral to hospital could no longer be avoided. A closer look at what home helps actually did confirms and amplifies this impression.

Although the home help's official duties were domestic—cleaning the house, doing the shopping and preparing a meal—many of them undertook nursing activities as well. An example was a widow of eighty-eight, living alone, who had been in failing health for two years. Her general practitioner was satisfied that her deterioration was merely due to old age, but when she was eventually admitted to hospital, where she died soon afterwards, she was found to be suffering from cancer. She had had the same home help for the whole two years. At the time of her referral the patient was bedfast and incontinent, and had been so for three months. During all that period the home help had come in at 9 a.m. each morning to find the patient cold, hungry and soaking in urine. She made breakfast, kindled the fire, then stripped the bed, washed the patient, changed her, applied powder and cream to her skin, put her on a 'bed-pan' (more precisely she used a large shallow dish, known in Glasgow as an 'ashet'), emptied it, washed the soiled linen by hand and hung it up to dry. Then she tidied the house, slipped out to the shops, cooked a light meal and fed the patient. She accomplished all this in three hours (she was paid for two). She returned every evening to give the patient another bite to eat, to make her warm, clean and comfortable, and to tuck her up for the night.

This case was extreme but not exceptional. More than one-half of the home helps caring for geriatric patients undertook duties which were other than purely domestic. Half of them assisted the patient in excretory functions, and in many cases this involved helping the patient on and off the toilet, commode or bed-pan. Several of them washed linen soiled with human excreta, and took fouled linen home to their own houses and washed it in their own domestic washing machines.

Why did so many of the home helps attending geriatric patients undertake these extra tasks? They were compassionate human beings, and responded to the needs of their clients, most of whom were far too ill and far too deprived to be manageable at home. Moreover, it was the enlightened policy of the Home Help Department to encourage them to give all the help that was needed. The home helps acted not merely as substitutes for a daughter but as substitutes for a hospital. They were all that stood between this group of patients and total deprivation, apart from the sporadic help of relatives and neighbours. The number of patients picked off the floor in the morning by the home help after lying all night following a fall is grim testimony to the value of their regular visits. The two or four hours of service given by the home helps had to cover a twenty-four-hour need. By means of their devoted work patients were enabled to survive outside hospital, who should really have been in hospital receiving the twenty-four-hour care that they required.

Of course, ours was not a survey of all home helps, only of the minority attending patients who were referred to the geriatric unit. Many other old people were doubtless adequately maintained at home by home helps, because their needs were less, but had this service not been available they might otherwise have had to be admitted to hospital or residential home.

Of the patients who were cared for at home by relatives in conditions of intolerable strain only 1 in 7 had a home help. If the strain was so heavy, why did so few take the opportunity of lightening it? One answer was given by the daughter of Mrs McMorrow, a seventy-seven-year old unstable and demented Parkinsonian patient, who lived with her daughter, son-in-law and grown-up grandchildren. 'What good would a home help be to me?' she asked. 'All she does is the cooking and cleaning, and that is no trouble to me—in fact, I enjoy it and I wouldn't want anyone else to do it for me.' It was suggested that the home help might at least look after the patient for a short time and allow the daughter to go out, or even to take a part-time job. 'My mother would never agree to that,' responded the daughter. 'She won't have anyone else in the house. She wouldn't let my sister near her when she used to come through for the day from Edinburgh. She has got it into her head that I am the only one who can take her to the toilet, and if I go out she just wets herself, and it's twice as much work for me when I get back. Besides,' she added, 'they would charge £5 a week for a home help, and where is my husband going to find money like that on his pay?'

This case exemplified three of the main reasons for the non-use of the home help service in cases of 'strain': unacceptability to the relatives, unacceptability to the patient, and cost of the service. There were, however, a few among the geriatric patients, and doubtless many more in the general community, who obtained some relief of strain by sharing the burden with the home help. One such patient was Mrs Cramond, who lived with her husband and an unmarried daughter and who had become progressively more demented over a period of years. The daughter went out to work, and Mr Cramond could just about manage his wife for a couple of hours in the morning, but was exhausted by the time that the home help bustled in at 1 p.m. She made the lunch, took Mrs Cramond to the toilet and watched her till 5 p.m. while the husband rested; he then had only half an hour to do until his daughter arrived home from the office to take over the evenings. It wasn't much of a life for them all, but the system worked.

In the survey of 250 people who died after the age of sixty-five, described in Chapter 13, the utilization of home helps followed a similar pattern. Only 1 in 9 of these old people enjoyed the services of a home help during their final illness at home, and of those who were helpless, incontinent or mentally abnormal for a month or longer before their death or final admission to hospital, only 1 in 5 had a home help.

The next most important of the domiciliary services was district nursing. This service was provided by the Glasgow District Nursing Association under a contractual arrangement with the Medical Officer of Health. The general practitioner could arrange, by means of a telephone call to a district office, for a nurse to call once a day, or even more often, to assist the family in dressing, bed-bathing, care of the skin and of the bowels and other appropriate nursing procedures. The district nurse also gave advice and arranged for the loan of equipment. 'I don't know how I could have carried on without the nurse,' said Mrs Stoller's aged sister. 'She helped me to turn her in bed, looked after her skin, changed her, made the bed and always left her so comfortable. Sometimes I used to hear my sister groaning in bed, she was so uncomfortable, and I couldn't lift her, she was too heavy for me. But I used to tell her "Soon the nurse will be here", and that seemed to ease her pain.'

The proportions of geriatric patients who used district nurses and home helps were similar, but the patterns of use of the two services were very different. There was no shortage of district nurses at the time of the surveys, but only 1 in every 3 patients of the 'strain' group used the service, and only 1 in 5 of the group with insufficient basic care. In the community sample of old people who died at home or who were ill at home before final admission to hospital, only 13 per cent used a district nurse, and even among those who were bedfast, incontinent or mentally disturbed for one month or longer at home only 18 per cent had a district nurse.

The district nursing service is initiated by a request from the general practitioner. Why then did so few of those who could have benefited from the service actually receive it? In some cases of 'insufficient basic care' the patient's first contact with the general practitioner was at the time of his referral to hospital, so there was no opportunity to introduce the home nursing service. In other cases the doctor may have felt—and this is speculation—that a necessarily brief visit from a nurse would have made little impression on the patient's total needs. This view gains some support from the finding of the much greater use of district nurses by patients who obtained adequate basic care from their families; in their cases the help given by the nurse supplemented rather than substituted for care from the family.

Home nursing consisted mainly of bed-bathing, changing and turning the patient, bed-making, care of the skin and attention to pressure areas. Nurses also took time to train relatives in home nursing techniques. Routine enemas for bowel clearance were given in a few cases. Commodes and wheelchairs (usually of outmoded design) were supplied to a few patients. The nurses worked like Trojans during their necessarily short visit, and left behind them a clean and comfortable patient who had benefited greatly from their attention. Nevertheless, a strong impression was gained that home nursing could have contributed much more than it did if some general practitioners had been more aware of its potential and if the nurses had had more time, more help and more specially designed equipment with which to extend their service to the patients.

A list of domiciliary services available to the elderly contains the names of many other services provided by Regional Hospital Boards, Local Authorities and voluntary organizations, but none of these made any significant contribution to the care of geriatric patients. Three of the 280 geriatric patients received Meals-on-Wheels on two days a week; one used the home laundry service; none had a night-sitter; none were helped by a Good Neighbour service; none attended a day hospital; a few had domiciliary physiotherapy, occupational therapy or chiropody; none attended luncheon clubs or day centres. These deficiencies of community care were due either to non-existence of the service (day hospitals, Good Neighbours), low provision (Meals-on-Wheels, laundry service, night-sitters, occupational therapy, physiotherapy, chiropody), low utilization of an adequately available service (home helps, district nurses), or non-relevance of the service to the patient's needs (luncheon clubs, day centres). There were obvious financial and staffing difficulties to explain some of these inadequacies, but there was also a lack of any mechanism for determining what were the real needs and for devising and providing services to meet them.

The major element of community care in the survey of Glasgow geriatric patients was not provided by the Government, the Local Authority or the Regional Hospital Board, and cost the country nothing. This was the help which patients received from neighbours, exemplified by the case of Mrs Bird, a pert shrill old lady of ninety-three, once a saver of souls in a local evangelical mission, but now living alone in a pensioner's flat. She was confined to bed with an undiagnosed abdominal ailment which was possibly malignant, although her emaciation might equally have been due to her ascetic refusal of food over many years. Her three children had long since been driven, by Mrs Bird's evangelical enthusiasm to emigrate to Canada, New Zealand and the London Borough of Tower Hamlets respectively, and Mrs Bird's sole (human) support was her neighbour and erstwhile convert Mrs Trainer, with whom she had a love-hate relationship of feverish intensity. Mrs Bird sang Mrs Trainer's praises to the doctor in prose of exquisite elegance, richly embellished with Biblical quotations, and then, in a trice, abused the same angelic creature with thunderous ferocity for failing to place the pillows as she liked them. Mrs Trainer accepted praise and blame alike with meekness and modesty. 'She was a good soul that one,' said Mrs Trainer. 'Many's the one that has cause to be grateful to her.' Now Mrs Bird had cause to be grateful to Mrs Trainer, for the latter slept in her own home but did little else there, camping out in Mrs Bird's home, cleaning it, shopping, cooking, lifting Mrs Bird onto and off the commode, washing her, setting her hair, adjusting her pillows, fetching her drinks, and responding instantly to every whim of that dying old lady (she had been dying for several years and the process was not yet complete when this report was written). It was well that Mrs Trainer had been drilled by her mentor in the concept of service to others, because Mrs Bird left her little time to look after herself.

Mrs Trainer was one of twenty-nine neighbours who were the sole or major support of ill old people among the 280 subjects accepted for the geriatric unit (see Tables 25 and 26, pp. 141 and 142), and whose care of the patient extended far beyond the ordinary good neighbourly service to include such necessary activities as cleaning up incontinence, giving and emptying bed-pans, stripping beds, laundering sheets and helping in the toilet. Eighteen other neighbours provided regular assistance of a less arduous nature, including housework, shopping and the preparation of meals for the patient, while neighbourly social visits and sporadic assistance were given in countless other cases.

Neighbourly help was related to the patient's environment. Of the patients who lived in old tenement houses with outside toilets, twice as many were helped by neighbours as was the case with patients in more modern houses. Neighbourly help, unlike the formal social services, was a twenty-four-hour service to the patient. It was flexible and could be fitted in with the neighbour's own daily activities. It was acceptable because it was based on a similarity of social background and on an unwritten code of reciprocity ('You would do the same for me'). Perhaps it should form the template on which organized community care for the aged is to be built.

It is widely agreed that housing plays a crucial role in the health and happiness of the elderly. Among the geriatric patients, however, this role was overshadowed by the far greater importance of medical factors and family structure. If bad housing itself had accelerated the referral of old people to the geriatric unit, it would have been expected that more geriatric patients than control subjects would have occupied poor housing. This was not the case (see Table 14, pp. 134-5); the same proportion in each group were badly housed. This finding came as no surprise to the doctor and the social worker. It was seldom that old people living in homes which lacked all basic amenities complained of the house; on the contrary, they held it, in many cases, in pathetic affection. 'It's ma ain wee hoose and ah wouldnae leave it,' said one old woman, surveying with pride her home of one room, three stairs up in an old tenement, with an outside toilet on the stairs. Of course, some patients complained bitterly that they could no longer reach the outside toilet, or that they could not go out to the shops because of the stairs, or that the house was damp and draughty, but just as many complaints were received from the occupants of new houses—they were too far away from relatives and friends, they couldn't get to the shops or to the bus, the neighbours were all out at work, they missed a coal fire, the electricity bills were huge, and so on. No one would deny the value of modern plumbing. The point to be made is that the ill old people in this survey attached as much or more importance to the human environment of their houses as to the physical environment. The impression was gained that insufficient attention had been paid to these aspects of environment in the earlier post-war housing schemes.

The finding that geriatric patients who lived in tenement houses with outside toilets received twice as much help from neighbours as did those who lived in modern houses with bathrooms (see Table 26, p. 142) can be explained in several ways. The tenement-dwellers had occupied their houses for twenty, thirty or forty years, or even longer. They had gone through life together with their neighbours, attending one another in childbirth and sharing the upbringing of children. The front doors of their houses were left open, and neighbours drifted in and out as though into rooms of the one house. The help provided to one another during illness was given naturally and unquestioningly. Amongst the better-housed patients fewer lived alone; many lived with family members and did not require the help of neighbours. Those in newer houses had not been there long, and there had not been time for the close relationships to develop which characterized the tenement-dwellers.

There is much new thinking about the housing of old people today, and we are to have in future far more grouped warden-service flatlets, a type of housing which did not really exist in the East End of Glasgow in 1967. This pattern of old people's housing has been highly successful in other parts of the country. The grouping of flats into compact and convenient units provides an economical focus for deploying home help and meals services. The availability of warden supervision protects the frail and the forgetful from hazard, but at the same time the flatlet-dweller does not lose his cherished sense of independence. However, our experience leads us to suspect that many old people will resist these blandishments and elect to stay where they are. For them a house is much more than a place to live in: it is a love-object full of the possessions and memories of a lifetime. Old people should not be severed from their love-objects; if this is to be avoided they must be properly housed long before they are old. How this might be done is discussed in the next chapter.

Some 2 per cent of the elderly population of Glasgow lived in residential homes, but only one of these homes, run by a voluntary religious organization, was located in the East End of the city, and none of the patients referred to in the study lived in a home. However, nearly 10 per cent of the patients referred to the geriatric service and not thought to be in need of admission were considered suitable for homes, as were a number of other patients after completion of their treatment in the geriatric unit. The attitude of those who were advised to apply for admission to Eventide Homes was a mixture of apprehension and resignation, well summed up in the comment of one old man, 'Oh well, if there is nothing else for it, I suppose I will just have to give it a try.' Residential homes make a valuable contribution to the care of old people, but are seen by the old who live outside them as a threat to their most highly prized possession, their independence. It may be added that those who go to live in them do not always retain this opinion.

The declared objective of community care is to keep old people in their homes where, it is assumed, they can be cared for more happily and more economically than in institutions. If community care is to be effective it must keep the right people out of the institutions, and it must do so without creating more misery than it prevents. The present surveys cast very considerable doubt on all these assumptions about community care, at any rate in the context of ill old people in the East End of Glasgow in 1967 where, admittedly, not all the components of community care were to be found. Community care consisted, first, of a corps of splendid home helps exceeding their official commitments in order to keep out of hospital ill and deprived old people who should never have been kept out of hospital; next, of a group of overwrought, harassed, exhausted wives, daughters and other relatives endangering the health and happiness of themselves and their families in order to keep out of hospital ill old people who should have been in hospital, and asking very little help in the execution of their task from the domiciliary services; next, of a group of neighbours labouring away without reward or recognition, but out of sheer humanity, helping to keep out of hospital more old people who should never have been outside hospital; and fourth, a band of devoted hard-working district nurses, making their own contribution to keeping out of hospital ill old people who should have been inside hospital.

Of course, this survey is not an over-view of the whole problem of community care and the deployment of the domiciliary services. But it does demonstrate that for one very large section of those in need, community care is no panacea. In the East End of Glasgow in 1967 many more people needed treatment in hospital than were able to receive it, and community care was a poor substitute. If the cavalcade of miseries which accompany the old person in the last years of his life is to be substantially reduced, then there must be both a massive increase in the provision of institutional care and sheltered housing and a radical reorganization and expansion of the domiciliary services.

16   'Something Must Be Done'

According to the Registrar General of Scotland, between the years 1971 and 1981 the number of people in Scotland aged between sixty-five and seventy-four is expected to increase by 22,000, those aged between seventy-five and eighty-four by 38,000 and those aged eighty-five and over by 5,000. At present the annual death rate in these three age groups is 45 per thousand for those aged between sixty-five and seventy-four, 97 per thousand for those aged between seventy-five and eighty-four, and 233 per thousand for those aged eighty-five and over. The figures in Chapter 13 give the average duration of stay in hospital per death in Glasgow in the period immediately preceding death as 49 days for those who died aged from sixty-five to seventy-four, 102 for those aged from seventy-five to eighty-four, and 146 for those aged eighty-five and over.

Let us assume that the Glasgow experience is typical of Scotland as a whole, and that the pattern of hospitalization, morbidity and mortality in 1981 remains the same as it was in 1968. We have, of course, no evidence either to support or refute these assumptions, which are made purely as a point of departure for a discussion of the implications of our findings. We can then calculate that merely to accommodate the increased population of old people in Scotland in 1981 in hospital for the period preceding their death would require an additional 1,800 hospital beds. The arithmetic is presented in Table 57 (p. 161). One-half of these new beds would be in psychiatric units, one-third in geriatric units and one-sixth would be acute medical or surgical beds. To staff them would require some ten additional consultants (half of them psychiatrists), supported by about fifty junior hospital doctors, 100 ward sisters, 100 staff nurses, some 500 enrolled nurses and a similar number of nursing auxiliaries. To these must be added ancillary laboratory, administrative, technical, engineering and domestic staff.

Let us further assume, again purely for discussion and without evidence either way, that the pattern of dependency and of utilization of domiciliary services preceding final hospitalization or death at home is the same for Scotland as a whole as it was in the smaller survey of Glasgow, and that it remains the same in 1981. We can then make similar calculations about the increased requirements of domiciliary services. These show that approximately 1,000 more old people will require a home help, and a similar number will use the district nursing service during final illness.

These estimates relate only to the provision of care during final illness, and take no account of the demands on hospital and community services at other times. Since one-quarter of our geriatric beds were occupied by patients who were not in final illness, the total required increase of geriatric beds will be about one-third more than the figure already given. A somewhat lower figure might apply to psychiatric units, a slightly higher one to medical and surgical units, and a substantially higher one to community services.

The figures thus give a rough estimate of what will be required in Scotland as a whole over the next ten years, in order to stand still. This is what must be found in order that in ten years' time the situation will be the same as it is today. The same proportion of old people will enter hospital for want of basic care at home, or because their relatives collapse under unbearable strain; the same proportion will die at home while waiting for a bed that is not there for them; or the same proportion will fall in their own homes and lie all night on the floor unattended. This is the price of staying where we are. This is what we have to do to prevent things getting worse. We have not started to count the cost of doing things better.

The situation in Scotland is more favourable than in many other parts of the United Kingdom. Scotland has more geriatric beds and more consultant geriatricians per head of population than has England and Wales, and the increase in the number of very old will be even greater in England and Wales than in Scotland.

These estimates are based on the assumption that circumstances will not change over the next ten years. But changes can be expected, of which some, but not all, will be beneficial. On the credit side there are certain to be major alterations in the administration of the National Health Service, in the organization of general medical practice, and in the education and deployment of nurses, which should lead to improved co-ordination and more efficient utilization of services. Occupational pension schemes and national superannuation will improve the purchasing power and, hopefully, the diet and health of the elderly. The new generation of old people may be healthier than their predecessors, and more of them will have benefited from pre-retirement training. The physical amenities of their homes will be improved. Diminution of atmospheric pollution may reduce the amount of respiratory illness. The number of people reaching old age may not be as high as the Registrar General predicted a few years ago. The rise in deaths from myocardial infarction, cancer of the lung and road traffic accidents in middle age has already exceeded expectations. However, other factors will increase the difficulty of finding resources to deal with old people. Hospital buildings will be ten years older, and the replacement of many of these is already long overdue. The post-war 'bulge' in the birth rate will have moved on, and the number of girls leaving school and becoming available to enter nursing and the other health professions will have fallen sharply. Advances in medical care, such as extension of intensive and coronary care units and of organ transplantation, will absorb more resources and man-power. Improvements in medical treatment will mean the graduation into old age of many disabled survivors of formerly fatal diseases. The prospect of finding a cure for the major disabling diseases of old age is slender. The volume of research into dementia and incontinence is pitifully small in proportion to the magnitude of the problems. Research into atherosclerosis is proceeding at a greater pace, but even if a drug was to be made available tomorrow which would arrest or reverse the disease, we would still be faced with the multitude of people whose tissues have been already damaged by its effects and with the formidable problems of social engineering necessary to bring the treatment to the patient. As long as dementia and incontinence remain unconquered, they threaten to nullify the gains made by the conquest of other diseases.

Given this bleak situation what then can be done? The answer is, a great deal. The size of the problem suggests many lines of action, which can be divided into three groups:

1. Things that can be done today that cost little or no money.
2. Things that should be done today that cost money.
3. Things that must be done today, whether they cost money or not.

Taking the last group first, the things that must be done today, regardless of cost, are education and planning. Ill old people will be dealt with more efficiently if the professional people who look after them are educated and trained to do so. At the time of our survey the first university chair in geriatric medicine in the United Kingdom had only just been established in Glasgow. There was only one chair in general practice at Edinburgh. There were no chairs in experimental or social gerontology. The vast majority of medical students completed their education without ever seeing a geriatrician or entering a geriatric unit. The same was true for almost all student nurses, and for many physiotherapists, occupational therapists, speech therapists and medical social workers. The higher education in the problems of old age received by directors of social services and administrators of Regional Hospital Boards was scanty in the extreme. The facilities for providing such education in British institutions of higher learning were minuscule. The amount of research being undertaken into the biology of ageing, the aetiology, prevention and management of senile dementia, incontinence and the other 'great disablers', was also small in amount although of excellent quality. Research and experimentation into the operation of health and social services for the elderly was more advanced, but even in this field the work done was small in comparison with what could be done. Since 1967 there have been improvements in the education and research fields, especially in the post-graduate in- struction of general practitioners, while in 1970 two further chairs of geriatric medicine were established at Manchester and South- ampton. However, unless there are further rapid strides forward the majority of doctors who will be practising in the year 1990 will have received no formal undergraduate training in geriatric medicine.

This irrational situation must be corrected as quickly as possible. The universities must give the lead; the training schools and colleges for nurses, ancillary workers, social workers and administrators must follow. 'Where there is no vision,' wrote King Solomon, 'the people perish.'

The other field in which action must be taken today is the creation of a total environment suitable for potentially frail old people. An important contribution can be made by a greatly increased provision of grouped warden-service flatlets, in such numbers that these can be made available when the need arises. We see this need when a patient has completed treatment in hospital but is not really fit to return to an unsatisfactory home. At this stage patients are usually still reluctant to accept the sacrifice of their independence, which they believe is entailed in admission to a residential home, but many would be grateful to be rehoused in the conditions of comfort and companionship which warden-service flatlets could provide. The ready availability of sheltered housing at this stage might shorten the stay in hospital of this group of patients and release hospital beds for others. No doubt there are other times in an old person's life when the move to a warden-service flatlet would be welcome, for example after bereavement. But grouped flatlets cannot be the only answer. To some the very fact that they are 'special' makes them unacceptable, and there are likely to be difficulties in recruiting enough of the right type of warden. A policy is also required for 'normal' housing which takes adequate account of the following implications of life in an ageing society.

Every elderly couple can expect to spend an average of one year during which at least one of them is physically or mentally frail or housebound. One of them will outlive the other and will occupy the house alone. Help will be required from outside sources—family, neighbours or social services—during this period. The longer a person lives in the house the better adapted he becomes to it, and the better his links with neighbours. Change will be resisted with increasing intensity as the years go by.

A number of policy points can be derived from these statements:
1. People should move into the house in which their old age will be spent while they are still young, ideally when their children leave home or marry, that is when they are in their fifties. The policy can be expressed by the phrase 'the way to house old people is not to house old people, it is to house not-old people'.
2. 'Old people's houses' should be occupied by old people for twenty-five years on average, that is one-third of the occupant's life. So they should be normal houses situated in normal groupings, not special houses. At the same time it should be normal for them to contain sensible architectural features, like power sockets at waist height, wide bathroom doors, fittings for hand rails beside the toilet, and the like, which make them easily adaptable to the needs of the frail and which are equally convenient for the fit. They should have at least two rooms.
3. Married children should be housed within easy reach, so that mutual interchange of services becomes an established pattern of interaction and remains as the foundation for help in illness.
4. House sizes within estates or in high blocks should always be mixed, so that people with different housing needs can be accommodated close to one another.
5. There should be easy and preferably traffic-free access to shops.
6. Community social services should be de-centralized so that in each housing aggregate home help and nursing services could be economically deployed.

These principles are well understood by some planning authorities, but one wonders how many of the houses being built today will pose problems of isolation and inaccessibility to the old people who will occupy them in fifty years' time.

Architects and planners must accept that almost every house built today is liable to be occupied for part of its life by someone who can only with difficulty get out of it or move around in it, or who is liable to fall in it. This should be kept in mind every time a sheet of paper is pinned to a drawing board.

The things which should be done today and which cost money are the erection of more buildings and the recruitment of more staff to serve the aged. There is tremendous activity in building hospitals, hostels, centres, clinics, clubs, homes and sheltered housing for the ill, the old and the frail, all over the country, well documented in the

1970 report of the Royal College of Physicians of Edinburgh. There is no doubt about the enormous efforts made and the tremendous improvement attained. But the gap between the best and the worst areas remains very wide, the expansion of domiciliary services lags far behind that of institutional services, shortage of trained staff is an almost universal complaint, and in very few places are the services sufficient for present needs, let alone for the greatly increased needs to be expected in the immediate future.

At the national level there is a very simple choice before us. Either we decide that we want to look after our old people properly, and we make the large allocation of money and personnel which such a decision entails, or we decide that we cannot really afford to do so, and we struggle along doing the best we can with inadequate resources. In a word, we decide to perpetuate the Mrs McGoldricks. This is a political decision and will be made by the politicians, who presumably interpret the will of the electorate. But whatever political decision is made, there will still be a need for the professionals to decide how to make the most effective use of the resources allocated to them. In this area there is a great deal that can be done today at little cost, by widely putting into practice ideas which have already been tried out and found to work, and of which the following are examples.

Research in Edinburgh, London and elsewhere has established that among the many causes of disability in old age a number stand out which are easily detected and which are amenable to treatment. These include subnutrition, anaemia, heart disease, muscle weakness, deafness, visual impairment, foot troubles and depression. Many of the victims of these diseases fail to seek help because of apathy, reluctance or fear. If an effort is made to go out and find these people, many of them accept investigation and treatment. A small but very significant proportion of them spend two or three weeks in hospital being restored to fitness, and can then be discharged well. They might otherwise have declined into a prolonged state of dependency at home, followed by a lengthy and perhaps unsuccessful attempt in hospital to restore them to independence. Anything which reduces the total pool of disability diminishes the burden of strain on relatives and the volume of unmet need, and frees institutional and domiciliary services for use by others.

Schemes of this nature can be initiated by general practitioners themselves, working with health visitors or district nurses, and in collaboration with the geriatric physician; or the initiative can come from the geriatric department. The first requirement is a doctor with vision, enthusiasm, perseverance and a high level of diagnostic skill. If young doctors realized the opportunities for the deployment of these gifts of personality which both general practice and geriatric medicine afford, perhaps recruitment to these branches of the profession would be in a healthier state than it is today. Next, the qualities of flexibility, co-operation and willingness to experiment must be present in the hospital administrators and the Local Authority's departments of health and of social work. Third, the department of geriatric medicine needs a properly staffed outpatient clinic and a day hospital. Fourth, there must be facilities to deal with the treatable pathology which is revealed, much of which relates to the eyes, ears, teeth and feet. Fifth, the scheme requires specially trained health visitors or district nurses to call on old people at risk (the very old, those living alone, the recently bereaved and those who have recently left hospital), and to assess their needs. To this list might be added old people who have home helps, and those who have applied to enter homes. And finally, the commitment of the general practitioner to the scheme is necessary to ensure that recommendations made by the geriatricians are carried out; for this the assistance of a district nurse or health visitor attached to the practice is highly desirable. A scheme along these lines which was pioneered in Edinburgh by Dr J. Williamson and his colleagues has not caused any notable increase in the work-load of the geriatric unit in the short term. The long-term benefits remain to be assessed. Successful projects were also described in an Irish general practice by Burns and in an Edinburgh practice by McNabola.

All these schemes were preceded by many years by the establishment in Rutherglen, near Glasgow, in 1955, by Dr W. F. Anderson and Dr Nairn Cowan, of the first joint consultative health centre for old people, run by the hospital and Local Authority services in conjunction. It was dedicated to the same aim of detecting physical, mental and social malaise in the ageing population at an early stage, when investigation and treatment hold out maximum promise for their eradication.

The expansion of health centres affords an excellent opportunity for the widespread introduction of schemes for the early detection and treatment of high-risk old people. The home visiting stage can be done by nursing staff attached to the health centre and the medical examination by a general practitioner of the group, while a consultant can visit the centre and see selected cases together with the practitioner. This collaboration ensures that only those patients who are likely to benefit from further investigation and treatment attend or are admitted to hospital.

Another pioneering activity for which Glasgow can claim credit, and which emphasizes positive health in old age and the prevention of disability, was the establishment of a Retirement Council offering courses of pre-retirement training. These ideas have since spread to many other parts of the country.

The many statutory and voluntary organizations which provide housing, food, and financial, social, educational and cultural benefits for the elderly also play a major part in the prevention and early detection of physical and mental disability. Activities along all these lines can be developed and extended everywhere.

Turning next to the situation inside the hospitals and in the community, the following are a few of the things that can be done.

In general hospitals geriatric physicians should be brought in at an early stage to advise on the management and rehabilitation of patients with conditions such as fractured neck of femur and stroke, so as to help reduce the burden of residual disability. In some places this has been done very successfully by the creation of special wards.

Psychiatric units admitting elderly patients with mental symptoms need full diagnostic facilities for the detection and treatment of physical illness, along lines pioneered in Dumfries and elsewhere. They also require close integration with geriatric units and community services. Psychogeriatric assessment units may have some part to play in this field. The use of day hospitals, hostels, boarding-out schemes and intermittent admission are essential, so that the enormously long periods of final hospital care of elderly dements can be shortened. At the same time families must be helped before the burden of strain becomes intolerable.

More district nurses should be attached to geriatric units for short 'refresher courses', and should be provided with modern equipment for use in the home. Health visitors should be deployed more extensively than at present among the elderly, both in the conventional way and in case-finding schemes on the Edinburgh pattern.

All medical students should accompany geriatric physicians on their domiciliary assessment visits to deepen their insight into the problems of ill old people and their families.

Additional post-graduate courses in geriatric medicine should be provided for general practitioners, hospital physicians and surgeons, nurses, physiotherapists, occupational therapists, social workers and administrators.

The working of the home help service deserves careful study. The home help service emerges from our researches as the big success of community care. Success, it is said, should be reinforced, and suggestions have been made by others about enlarging the range of the home help's activities and increasing her status. From our restricted experience in the East End of Glasgow we urge caution. Our guess is that if the home helps known to us were trained, put into uniforms, given professional status and told that they were vital members of the community care team, they would run away and never be seen again. The attraction of the job to many of them seems to be based on the opportunity of giving personal service on a direct one-to-one basis, without demanding of them that they carry responsibility. There is limited room for experiment to find additional ways of taking advantage of the home help's close bond with her client. Perhaps better use could be made of her time by the central organization of laundry, window-cleaning and household repairs, and possibly also of shopping and food preparation. The client's requirements could be noted by the home help, who could forward them to her supervisor as is the usual practice in many respects already; she in turn would arrange for the necessary service to be provided. Some of these tasks, notably shopping and repairs, could be allotted to members of a Good Neighbour service, clubs for retired people or voluntary and Church organizations, or to people recruited personally by the home help supervisor. The provision of meals, at present entrusted to the Meals-on-Wheels service or offered sporadically by neighbours, could also be initiated by a request from the home help to her supervisor, and routed through the Good Neighbour service to a person living nearby, who would be suitably recompensed. For laundry, contractual arrangements might be made with a local commercial laundry, or a Good Neighbour might be found willing to do the washing in her own domestic machine. One Good Neighbour with a car might be able to do the shopping for several home help clients, bringing in foods of the old person's own choice. She might visit and cook and serve the meal. In this way the old person would benefit by seeing more faces as well as by receiving more services. The home help could deal with more clients, and more members of the public would be involved in helping old people to live at home. The Good Neighbours themselves would be recruited from people with time on their hands, notably the 'young old'—retired people in the sixty-five to seventy-four age group, younger widows, even busy housewives. The flexibility of hours and the informal nature of the work might suit the needs of many people. The service could be economical, but need not depend solely on volunteers. A scale of payment could be devised, and the job might be very attractive to, for example, widows with young children who needed the money but who could not cope with an ordinary job.

The key figure in this domiciliary service is the area home help organizer. She is in close contact on the one hand with a group of home helps, and through them with their clients, and on the other hand with the area social worker, and through her with the social security officer and other welfare services. She also has contacts with the health visitor and the local general practitioners. The area organizer in turn comes under a chief organizer, who is a senior official of the Social Work Department. Home help organizers are trained specifically for their job, although they are not necessarily professionally qualified social workers. Home helps themselves are now receiving some in-service training, and are encouraged to seek out areas of unmet need and to report them for action.

The success of the Good Neighbour service in the London Borough of Camden and elsewhere encourages us to hope that a service along similar lines would be practicable and helpful in many urban areas. We have no direct knowledge of rural conditions, but we believe that something like this scheme tends to develop spontaneously in the villages and the countryside.

Community nursing, also, is at present undergoing a process of re-appraisal. Much of the work needed by ill old people at home, such as bed-making, bathing and changing, can be done by nursing auxiliaries working in pairs, with access to a laundry service. There is an increasing trend for nurses to work in teams consisting of health visitors, registered nurses, enrolled nurses, nursing auxiliaries and perhaps nurses in training; in many cases these teams are associated with health centres or group practices. The nurses have access to a pool of modern equipment, and have periodic refresher courses or study days in hospitals. More of the nurse's time is spent in training relatives and in supervising the loan of equipment. These desirable trends should be encouraged.

Relief must be provided to aged spouses, daughters and others enmeshed in the home care of the severely disabled and the mentally disturbed. The solutions usually proffered—paying the daughter as a home help, or providing a 'Granny-sitting' service—have, in our experience, only very limited application. Intermittent relief admission of the patient to hospital is not always acceptable, but could be practised more in the form of 'six weeks in–six weeks out', or for two weeks every three or six months, or for one day a week. Day hospital attendance is a great help in this respect, especially for the mentally frail. Our study suggests that one of the more effective methods of keeping a daughter from being overwhelmed by strain is to encourage her to go out to part-time employment. This might involve having a home help to look after the patient while the daughter worked to earn the money to pay for the home help. This situation is not quite so illogical as it seems, and a sympathetic and realistic scale of charges might be introduced in these circumstances.

Finally, a task which every authority should undertake, and which many already do, is to keep themselves informed of the nature and extent of the problem in the area for which they are responsible; to review constantly the efficiency of their services; to learn what is being done elsewhere that might be done in their area; and to keep the public and the policy-makers constantly aware of the needs which remain to be met. There seems to be ample scope for the larger Local Authorities to collaborate in these respects with university departments to their mutual benefit.

Many a time in the course of their work the doctor and the social worker standing in the house of one of the untended sick, knowing of the waiting list for admission to the geriatric unit and the insufficiency of community resources, have blanched to hear a worn-out neighbour say, 'Something will have to be done'. In this chapter, an attempt has been made to state what that 'something' is, and how much it will cost. The following words, taken from the 'Ethics of the Fathers' seem apt:

The day is short

And the work is great

And the Master of the House is urgent...

It is not required of you to complete the work,

But neither are you free to withhold yourself from it.

Part II

Materials and Methods; Definitions

A. Characteristics of the Area

The work described in this book was done in Glasgow in 1966–8, most of it in the eastern part of the city.

Table 1 (p. 126) presents population figures for 1966. Table 2 summarizes the hospital beds available, while Table 3 lists the domiciliary and residential services provided by the Corporation of Glasgow and by voluntary organizations, along with comparative figures for Scotland as a whole.

The work of the Department of Geriatric Medicine of the Glasgow Royal Infirmary Group during the three years of the study is summarized in Table 4.

B. Survey of Geriatric Patients

The main material on which this book is based is a survey of 612 people referred to the Department of Geriatric Medicine of the Glasgow Royal Infirmary Group of hospitals. These were routine cases, not specially selected in any way, and the patients were managed exactly as they would have been had there been no research project, except that their social circumstances were investigated in greater detail than is possible in ordinary working conditions.

The 612 referrals included thirty-nine subjects who were each referred twice, and one who was referred three times, that is there were 571 individuals in the series. However, since the object of this survey was to characterize the medical and social problems which led to the patients being referred to the geriatric unit, it was considered that the episode of referral rather than the individual was the unit to be studied. Throughout the report of the study the word 'subject' or 'patient' is used when, strictly speaking, 'referral' would be more accurate. The definitive study was preceded by a pilot investigation of fifty referrals, during which staff were familiarized with the procedures and methods were worked out.

The 612 subjects of the main survey were all those seen by one of the two physicians of the department, in the period 1 October 1966 to 31 December 1967. Of these patients 439 were referred from their own homes by their general practitioners, and 173 patients came from Glasgow Royal Infirmary or from one of the other hospitals in the group. All patients were seen by the geriatrician at home or in the referring ward within twenty-four hours of receipt of the request. He obtained the medical history, made a clinical examination, and assessed the patient's need for admission to the geriatric unit or for other services. The information was recorded on a form (see Appendix A).

The clinical data recorded about each patient included the presence and duration of strokes, falls, difficulty in walking, incontinence and mental abnormality. These were defined as follows:

1. *Stroke.* 'Recent major stroke' was defined as a loss of motor power in one or more limbs, with or without accompanying changes of perception, cognition and communication, presumed to be due to cerebrovascular disease, which was considered to be the major reason for the current referral to hospital.
2. *Falls.* Falls were recorded when the patient had suffered more than one fall indoors during a current or recent illness, or when a single fall had been followed by a period of lying helplessly on the floor, unable to rise until a helper arrived who had not been in the house at the time of the fall.
3. *Immobility.* This signified the inability of the patient to rise from his bed and to walk as far as the toilet in his own home without human support.
4. *Incontinence.* This was recorded in the presence of frequent or persistent incontinence of urine and/or faeces; isolated or irregular episodes were excluded.
5. *Mental abnormality.* The definition of mental abnormality used for the study was loss or severe impairment of the capacity for self-care and self-preservation, or the occurrence of socially unacceptable behaviour, as a result of adverse intellectual or emotional change. The abnormality was of such severity as to be clearly discernible to the relatives as being due to mental disease. Most cases of mental abnormality were dementia, some were acute confusional states, and a few were severe depressions.

Information about each patient referred from home was passed to a social worker, who visited the patient at home, interviewed him and his relatives, and built up a picture of the patient's domestic and social background, of the impact of his illness on the relatives, and of the response of the family and friends and the social services to the patient's needs. The relatives of patients seen in hospital were also interviewed by the social worker. The form used for the social worker's report is given in Appendix B.

The fate of every patient referred to the study was recorded twelve months after the date of referral under three headings: 'at home', 'in hospital', or 'dead'. In addition, those patients who were actually admitted to the geriatric unit were reviewed three months after the date of admission, and were classed under the headings: 'discharged home', 'still in hospital', or 'dead'. This classification referred to the immediate outcome of hospitalization, so that patients were classified as 'discharged' if they left hospital, even if they subsequently died or were re-admitted within the three-month period.

The items recorded by the doctor and the social worker were of three types—facts, recollections and value-judgments. The facts, such as the patient's marital status or whether the house had a bathroom, were straightforward. Information about the presence and duration of symptoms, which relied on the comprehension and recollection of the subjects and their relatives, was more liable to error and uncertainty. The social worker and the doctor had to judge the accuracy and motivation of each informant, and to seek independent corroboration from the general practitioner. To reduce the effect of errors of recollection only broad time-scales were used. Questions requiring value-judgment were the following:

1. What was the probable outcome of treatment in hospital—early death, discharge or prolonged retention in hospital?
2. For what reason was the patient accepted for the geriatric unit?
3. Did the patient receive sufficient basic care at home, and if not why was this?
4. Did the relatives experience undue strain in caring for the patient, and if so why?

At a weekly meeting of the research group these questions were posed in respect of all patients seen in the previous week. Initial difficulties in reaching agreement were traced to the following causes:

1. Difference in the information possessed by different members of the group.
2. Differences of interpretation of the agreed definitions.
3. Differences in the attitude of the observers to the patient's situation.
4. Differences in the assessment of the sincerity of the subjects and their relatives.
5. Differences in interpretation of how the family unit behaved before the patient's illness.

106

Once the main study was under way, disagreement about classification was rare, and was easily resolved by discussion. Nevertheless, it remains unavoidable that many of the conclusions of the survey depended on the subjective evaluation by fallible observers of subtle and elusive situations. The possibility of error is readily admitted, but every effort was made to be fair, reasonable and consistent.

Studies were made of various sub-groups of the original 612 geriatric patients. These included 173 patients referred to the geriatric unit from other hospitals in the group (Table 5), 53 patients accepted for admission who were under the age of sixty-five at the time of referral (Table 6), 21 patients selected for referral to the psychiatric unit (Table 7), and 14 patients thought to be in need of admission to Local Authority residential homes.

The remaining part of the analysis of geriatric patients related to those patients who were seen at home and who were accepted for admission to the geriatric unit. There were 280 in this group, of whom 25 were under the age of sixty-five. The analysis dealt with the presence and duration of symptoms of dependency, the reason for acceptance to the unit, and the outcome of treatment (Tables 8–11).

C. The Control Group

For every one of the 612 patients in the main survey a 'control' was selected by taking at random from the list of the patient's general practitioner the name of another person of the same sex as the patient and in the same five-year age group.

Method

Each month a list was sent to the Executive Council of the City of Glasgow, and to the councils of adjacent areas when appropriate, containing the name, sex, age and general practitioner of every patient referred to the study, either from home or from hospital, during that month. The Executive Council was asked to furnish the name of an appropriate control subject, the initial letter of whose surname most closely followed that of the patient. If there was no other person on the general practitioner's list in the same age and sex group (and this happened in a few instances, mainly with males over the age of eighty), a name was taken from the list of the general practitioner whose practice was closest to that of the patient's own doctor. In a few instances the control subject proved to be a patient who was himself in the main survey, but this did not prevent his use as a control for another patient. Nine other control subjects proved to be in hospital or in a residential home; these subjects were also included. The forty individuals who were referred more than once

107

in the main survey were allocated the same control subject at each referral. The names and addresses obtained from the Executive Council were then checked with each general practitioner's receptionist. Those which referred to patients who had died or moved away from the district were removed from the list, and the Executive Council provided a new name in place of these. Circular letters (see Appendix C) were then sent to each general practitioner explaining the purpose of the survey and asking for his permission for the subject to be interviewed. Only one general practitioner objected. Controls for this doctor's patients were obtained from nearby practitioners. The remainder readily agreed to the social worker's visit. Some general practitioners notified the subjects that the social worker would be calling. The other subjects were visited without previous notification. The vast majority welcomed the interview and readily gave all the information required. The same data sheet was used by the social workers as was used in the main survey.

Despite the assurances given to them a few control subjects expressed anxiety or perplexity. Some of the more confused resented or misunderstood the social worker's visit and thought that it was connected with rehousing, pensions, social security, or admission to a residential home. One patient's daughter telephoned the department in indignation, saying that her mother had no wish or need to enter a residential home. Such incidents were rare; the vast majority enjoyed being visited and questioned. The investigators often found it difficult to get away from the house, and were pressed to return for another chat.

Many subjects were out when the investigators called, and repeat visits had to be made. In a few instances, the information was provided by relatives or neighbours, but there seemed no need to doubt its accuracy in these cases.

In Table 12 the age distribution of the geriatric patients and their controls is compared with that of the population as a whole. Tables 13 and 14 present a comparison between the social characteristics of the geriatric patient and the control group, while Table 15 lists difficulties encountered in interviewing the control subjects.

D. The 'Medical' Control Group

In order to determine how geriatric patients differed from old people admitted to general medical wards, a survey was carried out, with the co-operation of the physicians of Glasgow Royal Infirmary, of 250 patients aged sixty-five and over admitted to the beds during two observation periods, one in the winter of 1967 and one in the summer of 1968. These were unselected consecutive admissions of older patients to the medical wards. The information obtained about these patients included age, sex, marital status, social indices and the presence and duration, in the period preceding admission, of the symptoms of dependency. The same data sheet was used for this survey as in the main survey. Each acute medical ward was visited weekly, and all patients aged sixty-five and over admitted in the previous week were studied. When patients were unable to give the required information because they were too ill, confused, deaf or aphasic, or because they died soon after admission, a home visit was paid and the relatives' help was enlisted.

A comparison was then made of the age and social and medical factors of the geriatric patients with that of the elderly 'medical' patients. The geriatric patients were the 255 subjects already described who were aged sixty-five and over and who were referred from their own homes and accepted for admission to the geriatric unit. The comparisons are presented in Tables 16 to 20, and the results are discussed in Chapter 4.

Quality of Care

The quality of care received by the geriatric patients is described in Chapters 8 to 14. In this part of the study, data were analysed for the 280 patients who were seen at home and accepted for admission to the geriatric unit. They were classed as receiving 'sufficient' or 'insufficient' basic care, as defined in Chapter 6, and as receiving this care with or without 'undue strain'. The characteristics of these groups are shown in Tables 21 to 23 and 31 to 33. Tables 24 to 26 list the help given by relatives and neighbours, and Tables 27 to 30 and Table 34 show the use made of the domiciliary social services.

E. The Incontinence Survey

The small study of incontinence, described in Chapter 14, was based on data obtained from the survey of geriatric patients. Among the last 100 patients referred, there were twenty who had been persistently incontinent at home for two days or longer at the time of their referral. A special questionnaire (Appendix D) was prepared, on which were recorded detailed information about the measures used to manage the symptom of incontinence. This material is described in Chapter 14 and the data are recorded in Table 35.

F. Survey of Final Illness

The survey of final illness, which is described in Chapter 13, took place in two parts. In the larger survey an analysis was made of all deaths which occurred of people normally resident in the City of

Glasgow who died in Scotland during the year 1968 and who were aged sixty-five years or over at the time of death. No information was available about deaths which occurred outside Scotland of persons normally resident in Glasgow. For those deaths which took place in hospital, information was obtained about the duration of terminal stay in hospital and the type of ward in which the patient was cared for. A note was also made of the age, sex, marital status and social class of the subject, the last of these being determined by the main occupation of the patient or spouse, as recorded in the death certificate (Registrar General's Classification of Occupations, 1966). The information was complete except for fourteen deaths which occurred in one nursing home. The management committee of this home felt that it would be a breach of confidentiality for them to give access to their case records to the investigators, so it was not possible to record for these subjects the source of admission and duration of terminal stay in that nursing home.

Methods

In Scotland death is registered in the parish in which it occurred, and a copy of the registration certificate is sent to the registrar of the parish in which the deceased normally resided. The information given includes the name, usual address, sex, age, occupation and place of death of the deceased. In Glasgow in 1968 this information was retained in the Registration Section of the Health and Welfare Department. All the certificates for 1968 were scrutinized and, for those persons who were aged sixty-five and over at death, the necessary information was entered on a form (Appendix E). For deaths which occurred in a hospital each hospital was visited in turn, the records were studied and information was recorded about the ward in which death occurred, the duration of stay in hospital and transfers from one ward to another. Hospital wards were classified into four categories: medical, surgical, geriatric and psychiatric.

Nursing homes were those registered with the Corporation of Glasgow under the National Assistance Act, 1948. The term nursing home also included a Roman Catholic Hospice for the Dying, and a home for terminal cancer cases run by the Marie Curie Foundation.

Subjects Admitted before the Age of Sixty-five

Forty-eight patients who died at the age of sixty-five or over, after spending more than one year in hospital, were admitted before the age of sixty-five, as shown in the following table:

| Type of ward | Age on admission | | | | |
| | Number in age group | | | | |
	Under 30	30–49	50–9	60–4	Total
Medical/surgical	0	0	0	0	0
Geriatric	0	0	1	3	4
Psychiatric	7	16	7	14	44

If the total period of stay in hospital of the forty-four psychiatric patients who were admitted before the age of sixty-five is included in the calculation of the average duration of terminal stay of all patients in psychiatric wards, then a figure of six years is obtained. If this group of patients is excluded from the calculation, the average duration of stay of the remaining psychiatric patients is only two years. Neither of these courses seems justifiable. The very prolonged stay of these patients reflects past admission policies, and they did not necessarily need full mental hospital care throughout their stay, but might well have required this in the later part of their lives. For the calculation of average stay used in the study, the compromise was made of taking as the period of terminal stay of these forty-four patients the interval between the sixty-fifth birthday (or, when the birthday was unknown, 1 July in the year in which the age of sixty-five was reached) and death. All forty-four of these patients died before the age of seventy-five. By this method of calculation the average duration of stay in a psychiatric hospital for all patients was two and three-quarter years. For the four patients admitted before the age of sixty-five who died in a geriatric ward the total duration of stay in hospital was recorded.

Transfers

During terminal hospitalization 362 patients were transferred from one type of ward to another. In this group the place of death was recorded as that in which death actually occurred, but the total days spent in hospital were appropriately apportioned between the different types of unit in which the patient had been treated. The denominator in the calculation of average duration of stay in the various types of ward was thus 'episodes of stay' not 'patients'.

Results

The results of this large survey are given in Tables 36 to 48.

G. Retrospective Study of Final Illness

A more detailed survey was made of a small sub-sample of the main series. Information was sought about the nature and duration of symptoms during the final illness at home. This was obtained both for subjects who died at home, and for those who died in hospital, and the questioning of the latter group centred on the care required at home in the period preceding final admission to hospital. Information was also obtained about the provision of care by relatives and the use of domiciliary social services.

Material and Methods

The subjects of this survey were all who died in the period 1 January to 29 February 1968, who were aged sixty-five or over at the time of death and who normally resided in the eight electoral wards which form the east and south-east postal districts of Glasgow.

There were 260 deaths recorded. Ten which occurred in ambulances or public places were not further considered. In ten more cases relatives were unwilling to answer the interviewer's questions. There remained 240 subjects, of whom 106 died at home and 134 in hospital. In all these cases sufficient information was obtained from surviving relatives and other sources for the purpose of the study.

The use of only one part of the city and one period of the year was made necessary because the interviewers were available for only a short time, and it was desirable to reduce their travelling time and to ensure that the interval between the subject's death and the interview with relatives was neither too short nor too long.

A comparison between the sub-sample and the main sample is presented in Table 49.

Procedure

The procedure followed for tracing relatives of the deceased and obtaining interviews with them was as follows. The address of the next of kin was obtained from the death certificate. A letter was then sent to the relatives (see Appendix F) explaining the survey and indicating when the interviewer would like to call. If no informant could be found at the address or the practitioner was unable to help, a visit was paid to the patient's last recorded address. A relative was sometimes contacted in this way; otherwise a neighbour or a local shopkeeper was able to give the address of a relative, or, in a few cases, to furnish the required information himself. When these resources failed, approaches were made to the home help department, the Corporation Housing Department, the district nursing service, the local minister or anyone else who might be able to help. The experience of the interviewers in contacting their sources of information is summarized in Table 50. The data sheet used is shown in Appendix G.

The duration of symptoms, especially of mental abnormality, was not always accurately recollected by relatives. To minimize errors this information was checked from other sources whenever possible, and was classed only in broad categories. In Tables 51 to 56 are presented data concerning age, sex, social and medical factors, place of death, help received and use of social services by the subjects in this survey.

Projections

In Chapter 16 reference was made to the projected future need of hospital beds and of domiciliary services in Scotland. The calculations on which the argument was based are shown in Table 57.

Appendices

APPENDIX A Medical Data

Patient's name   Age   Serial number

Home address   Telephone number

General practitioner's name and address   Telephone number

Relatives' names and addresses, etc.

Date of doctor's visit   Date of social worker's visit

Source: home/residential home
         hospital — medical
                 surgical
                 psychiatric
                 other

Symptoms (see definitions)

Stroke: none	Falls: none
old	single, with long lie
recent minor	multiple, no long lie
recent major	multiple, with long lie

Ambulation: independent	Incontinence: none
unstable	infrequently
dependent	incontinent
helpless	frequently incontinent

                          Mental state: normal
                                      abnormal

Number of <u>major</u> symptoms (only categories underlined constitute <u>major</u> symptoms):

Longest duration of any <u>major</u> symptom: 6 days or under
7–28 days
29 days to 3 calendar
    months
3–6 months
6–12 months
more than 1 year

Care required: no inpatient care
basic care
medical/nursing
rehabilitation

For those accepted, reason for acceptance: therapeutic optimism
medical urgency
basic care
relief of strain

For those not accepted, recommendation:
outpatient treatment
domiciliary treatment
refer to general hospital unit
refer to psychiatric unit
refer to Corporation Welfare Dept.
terminal illness

Prediction: likely to be discharged within 3 months of admission
likely to die within 3 months of admission
likely to be still in hospital 3 months after admission

Time on waiting list: 6 days or under
7–28 days
29 days to 3 calendar months
more than 3 months

Outcome 3 months after referral: still on waiting list
admitted to geriatric unit
admitted elsewhere
withdrawn before bed available
refused bed when offered
died on waiting list

Follow-up 3 months after admission: discharged
died
still in

Follow-up 1 year after referral: at home
died at home
in hospital
died in hospital

APPENDIX B Social Data

Sex: male
     female

Marital status: single
              married
              widowed, separa-
              ted or divorced

Age: under 60
     60–4
     65–9
     70–4
     75–9
     80–4
     85–9
     90 and over

Social class: I and II
            III
            IV
            V
(Registrar General's classification)

Housing: Corporation pensioners' flatlets ⎱ both with bath and
         other Corporation house   ⎰   WC
         other house (not Corporation) with bath and WC
         other house with inside WC but no bath
         other house with outside WC only
         hostel (lodging-house)
         other (specify)

Number of living children:

Number of locally resident children:

Living arrangements: alone
                 with spouse only
                 other one-generation (brother/sister/friend)
                 with unmarried/widowed child only
                 other two-generation
                 three- or four-generation
                 other household (specify)

Help received from: spouse
              daughters/sons   (Indicate type of
              other relatives   help received using
              friends or neighbours   code below.)
              Corporation home help
              employed help

Type of help: 0 not available
            1 no help
            2 domestic only
            3 personal
            4 aid with toilet
            5 intimate cleansing

Chief helper: spouse   Chief helper's age: under 30
            child   30–49
            child-in-law   50–69
            sister/brother   70 and over
            other relative
            non-family   Chief helper's sex: male
                                                        female

Stayed off work to provide sufficient care: no one
                                                spouse
                                                son
                                                daughter
                                                other

Basic care received: insufficient
                            sufficient, no strain on helpers
                            sufficient, undue strain

If basic care is unsufficient, indicate lack: warmth
                                              cleanliness
                                              food
                                              safety

Reason for non-provision of care: no family
                                    preoccupation
                                    dilemma
                                    refusal
                                    neglect

Preoccupation: necessary employment
                     inadequate housing
                     own ill health
                     similar prior commitment
                     incompatible personalities

Dilemma: employment
            overcrowding
            family well-being
            personality difficulties

If sufficient care is provided only at cost of undue strain, indicate factors causing strain:

Factors in the patient: physical   Factors in the helper: physical
                       mental   mental
                       personality   person-
                       environmental   ality

Factors in the helper's life-space: employment
                                         housing
                                         finance
                                         care of other invalid
                                         care of young children
                                         loss of living space
                                         family relationships
                                         conjugal relationships
                                         loss of social life

Meals-on-Wheels: no
                      yes

District nurse: no
                   less than once daily
                   once daily at least

Home help ... number of hours per week:

District nurse ... number of visits per week:

Meals-on-Wheels ... number of meals per week:

Other domiciliary services (specify):

APPENDIX C Circular letter to General Practitioners

Dear Doctor,

With the assistance of the Scottish Home and Health Department this Unit is studying in detail the social and medical circumstances of patients referred to the Geriatric Service. To give us a perspective of the problem we need information about the family structure and housing conditions of people of the same age group and roughly the same background as the patients. We have therefore asked the Executive Council to draw at random from the list of each General Practitioner who refers a patient to the Unit the name of another patient in the same age group to serve as a Control. Our Social Worker would like to interview these control subjects and obtain the required information. No questions about the medical conditions of the control subject will be asked.

Your patient ... ... was recently referred to the Unit, and the control subject selected by the Executive Council is ... ... Our Social Worker would like to call shortly and if you have any comments or if for any reason you would prefer her not to call I hope you will get in touch with me.

Yours sincerely,

etc.

APPENDIX D   Incontinence

How long frequently incontinent of urine:
          infrequently incontinent of urine:
          frequently incontinent of faeces:
          infrequently incontinent of faeces:

Present ambulation status:

Duration of any dependence of ambulation:

Who cleanses patient?   self
Who empties commode, bed-pan, etc.?   spouse
Who washes soiled linen?   resident, same sex
                                                resident, opposite sex
                                                non-resident family
                                                non-resident non-family
                                                Corporation home help
                                                district nurse
                                                other (specify)

How many times is patient cleansed on average, by day:
                                          by night:

How long does cleansing take:

Where is WC?   inside, no stairs   outside, no stairs
                inside, stairs   outside, stairs

Does patient have incontinence pads?   yes, from NHS
                    plastic sheets: yes, from voluntary
                    commode: organization
                    bed-pan: yes, purchased
                    urinal: no

How are incontinence pads disposed of: burned indoors
                                        flushed down toilet
                                        placed in dustbin
                                        other disposal (specify)

Where is soiled linen washed:
    patient's home   laundrette
    family member's home   laundry
    non-family member's home   public wash house
    home help's home   Local Authority Home
                                        Laundry Service

Source of hot water: immerser
                     coal fire
                     no hot water supply

121

Number of sinks:

Washing machine: yes
                 no

First-stage drying facilities: none
                            hand-wringer
                            automatic wringer or spin-drier

Second-stage drying: none
                    overhead pulley
                    drying cabinet
                    tumbler drier
Summarize laundering procedures: done at home, adequate
                                    facilities
                             done at home, inadequate
                                    facilities
                             done away from home

Average number of soiled items washed daily:

Average time devoted to laundering daily:

Average weekly cost (estimated):

Was financial assistance with laundry received from Ministry of Social Security:

Are helpers aware of Local Authority Home Laundry Service:

District nurse: yes
                no

Health visitor: yes
                no

APPENDIX E   Survey of Final Illness

Name   Serial number

Address

Date of death

Sex: male   Age:
　　 female   (date of birth)

Marital status: single
　　　　　　　 married
　　　　　　　 widowed, separated or divorced

Occupation:
(for social classification according to Registrar General)

Place of death: home   medical ward
　　　　　　　 public place   surgical ward
　　　　　　　 ambulance   geriatric ward
　　　　　　　 on holiday   psychiatric ward
　　　　　　　 residential home   nursing home

If death was in hospital or nursing home, record:

Total number of days spent consecutively in hospital prior
　　 to death:

Number of transfers from one unit to another during this
　　 period:

Dates of all transfers:

Divide total days spent in hospital (or nursing home) into
　　 the following categories:

　　　　　 days in medical ward
　　　　　 days in surgical ward
　　　　　 days in geriatric ward
　　　　　 days in psychiatric ward
　　　　　 days in nursing home

APPENDIX F   Letter to Bereaved Relatives

Dear ... ...

A great deal of work is being done at the moment planning for the needs of people over the age of sixty-five. We are endeavouring to collect information from the relatives of people who have recently died and wonder whether you would be prepared to help us.

A member of our team will call on you in the near future to ask a few questions about the late ... ... whose name appears on the list supplied to us by the Registrar's Office at Martha Street.

We would be most grateful indeed to have your co-operation in this survey.

Yours sincerely,
SOCIAL WORKER

APPENDIX G   Dependency Survey

Name   Age   Serial number

Home address   Telephone number

Place of death   Date of death

Certified cause of death

General practitioner's name, address and telephone number
Information from hospital records:

    Name of hospital: Unit number:

    Date of admission:

    Duration of stay:

    Type of ward in which death occurred:

If patient was transferred from other hospital to hospital in which death occurred, record:

    Name of other hospital: Unit number:

    Date of admission:

Total duration of continuous hospital stay before death:

Information on social services: home help
                          health visitor   number of
                          district nurse   visits and
                          Meals-on-Wheels   duration, etc.
                          other

Home visit or consultation with general practitioner:

Date of interview:

Name of informant(s):   Relationship to patient:

Did informant live with patient?   Estimate accuracy of
                                        information:

With whom did patient live?

Relationship of principal helper to patient:

Age of principal helper (estimated):

Did patient have locally-resident child(ren)?

Duration of dependent ambulation:

Duration of incontinence:

Duration of mental abnormality:

Tables

Table 1 Population figures, 1966 (10 per cent sample census)

	Total population	Aged 65 and over	
		Number	Percentage
City of Glasgow	976,540	101,890	10
Eight eastern wards	247,570	22,600	9
Scotland	5,225,300	590,460	11
England and Wales	47,985,000	5,902,150	12

Table 2 Hospital beds, Glasgow, 1968

Medical[1]	3,186
Surgical[1]	2,715
Geriatric	1,813
Psychiatric[2]	4,853
Nursing homes[3]	325
Total[4]	12,892

Notes [1]Some of these beds were used by patients living outside the city boundary.
[2]Most of these beds were in hospitals located outside the city boundary which catered mainly but not exclusively for residents of Glasgow.
[3]These were beds in private nursing homes which were leased by the Western Regional Hospital Board for National Health Service patients.
[4]Equivalent to thirteen beds per thousand of the population excluding obstetric and paediatric beds.

(Source: Western Regional Hospital Board Annual Statistics, 1967–8)

Table 3 Domiciliary and residential services, 1968

Community service	GLASGOW	Per thousand of population	SCOTLAND	Per thousand of population
Residential homes (Local Authority)	1,841 places	1·8	8,018 places	1·5
Home helps*	1,101	1·1	5,005	0·95
District nurses*	158	0·17	901	0·17
Health visitors	210	0·22	1,174	0·22
Meals-on-Wheels per day	124	0·12	1,868	0·37

*Expressed in full-time equivalents.

(Sources: Annual Report Medical Officer of Health, Glasgow; Annual Report Health and Welfare Services in Scotland; Western Regional Hospital Board Annual Statistics)

Table 4 Glasgow Royal Infirmary, Department of Geriatric Medicine

	1966	1967	1968
Number of beds	308	355	474
Referrals: from home	778	695	872
from hospital	261	298	356
Total	1,039	993	1,228
Accepted for admission	735	698	842
Admitted	592	519	762
Admitted within one week	228	132	349
Died before admission	65	65	57
Admitted elsewhere	22	35	21
Discharged	311	238	370
Died in hospital	246	243	281
Number on waiting list on 31 December	37	44	61

(Additional information is available in the annual reports of the department.)

Table 5 Age and sex distribution and social and medical characteristics of patients referred from other hospitals

Age group	Male	Female	Total
Under 65	12	24	36
65–74	18	31	49
75–84	26	43	69
85 and over	5	14	19
Total	61	112	173

Social characteristics	Number	%
Married	40	23
Single	50	29
Widowed	83	48
No children in locality	98	57
Lived alone	73	42
With spouse only	32	19
With others	68	40
House with bathroom	95	55
House with WC but no bath	32	19
House with no WC and no bath	46	27

Medical characteristics	Number	%
Stroke	69	41
Immobility	132	76
Falls	43	25
Incontinence	67	40
Mental abnormality	83	48
Number of symptoms: one	29	17
two	41	24
three	54	31
four	24	14
five	5	3
none	20	11
Duration of dependency:		
less than one week	71	41
one week to one month	20	11
one month to one year	35	20
more than one year	25	14
not dependent	22	13
Number accepted for admission	136	78
Reasons for acceptance:		
therapeutic optimism	32	19
medical urgency	46	27
basic care	32	19
relief of strain	26	15
Number actually admitted	87	50
Outcome one year after referral:		
at home	19	11
in hospital	37	21
dead	30	17
untraced	1	0·6

Table 6 Patients accepted for the geriatric unit who were under sixty-five years of age

From home	25	Male	20
hospital	28	Female	33

Social and medical characteristics of those referred from home only

Male	13	Stroke	4
Female	12	Immobility	17
		Falls	8

129

Married	12		Incontinence		8
Single	5		Mental abnormality		9
Widowed	8				
			Number of symptoms: one		11
Lived alone	8			two	7
With spouse only	7			three	4
With others	10			four	1
				five	1
No local children	12			none	1

Outcome—three months after admission:

			Duration of dependence:	
discharged	11		less than one week	5
dead	2		one week to one month	1
still in hospital	8		one month to one year	6
not admitted	4		more than one year	9
			not dependent	4

Outcome—one year after referral:

at home	6
dead	12
in hospital	7

Table 7 Social and medical characteristics of twenty-one patients referred to psychiatric units[1]

Source: home	17		Stroke	0
hospital	4		Immobility	1
			Falls	4
Male	5		Incontinence	0
Female	16		Mental abnormality	21
Under 65	2		Duration of mental abnormality:	
65–74	6		less than one month	1
75–84	8	} all female	one month to one year	10
85 and over	5		one to five years	8
			more than five years	2
Married	4			
Single	4		Outcome—three months after	
Widowed	13		referral:	
			admitted to psychiatric	10
Lived alone	10		still at home	7
With spouse only	3		admitted to geriatric[2]	2
With others	8		unknown	2

130

Insufficient basic care	8
Sufficient with strain	9
Sufficient, no strain	4

Notes [1]These patients were referred originally by their doctors to the geriatric unit, but were considered by the geriatrician, after he had assessed the patient at home or in the referring unit, to require further care in a psychiatric unit.
[2]These cases, although recommended for psychiatric management, were admitted to the geriatric unit because no other accommodation was available. One was subsequently transferred to the psychiatric unit four months later. The other died soon after admission.

Table 8   Social characteristics related to reason for acceptance

Social characteristics	Therapeutic optimism	Medical urgency	Insufficient basic care	Relief of strain
Male	44	10	18	41
Female	61	9	49	48
Under 65	12	1	1	11
65–74	30	4	17	14
75–84	54	14	31	42
85 and over	9	0	18	22
Married	27	9	7	27
Single	18	3	12	9
Widowed	60	7	48	53
No children in locality	34	5	38	21
Lived alone	37	3	42	6
With spouse only	25	6	6	20
With others	43	10	19	63
House with bathroom	57	14	35	62
House with WC but no bath	23	2	17	13
House with no WC and no bath	25	3	15	14
Social class I and II	8	0	3	6
III	32	9	17	37
IV and V	65	10	47	46
Home help	24	2	36	14
District nurse	22	6	16	28
Meals-on-Wheels	1	0	2	0
Total	105	19	67	89

Table 9 Medical characteristics related to reason for acceptance

Medical characteristics	Therapeutic optimism	Medical urgency	Insufficient basic care	Relief of strain
Stroke	19	7	2	15
Falls	39	8	38	45
Immobility	54	19	46	76
Incontinence	20	8	31	49
Mental abnormality	37	9	32	56
Number of symptoms:				
one	39	3	11	20
two	27	5	24	17
three	16	7	23	22
four	7	3	4	24
five	0	1	1	5
none	16	0	4	1
Duration of dependency:				
less than one week	19	7	6	11
one week to one month	16	3	8	10
one month to one year	22	5	28	35
more than one year	25	4	20	28
not dependent	23	0	5	5
Total	105	19	67	89

Table 10 Reason for acceptance of geriatric patients aged sixty-five and over referred from their own homes

Reason for acceptance	Geriatric patients Number	%
Therapeutic optimism	93	36
Medical urgency	18	7
Basic care	66	26
Relief of strain	78	31
Total	255	100

Table 11 Reason for acceptance related to outcome

Reason for acceptance	Outcome—three months after admission									Total
	Discharged % of:			Died % of:			Still in hospital % of:			
	Number	Column	Row	Number	Column	Row	Number	Column	Row	
Therapeutic optimism	37	67	52	14	23	20	20	28	28	71
Medical urgency	3	5	23	5	8	39	5	7	39	13
Basic care	5	9	11	12	19	26	29	40	63	46
Relief of strain	10	18	17	31	50	53	18	25	31	59
Total	55			62			72			189

Table 12 Age distribution of geriatric patients and of the population as a whole

Age group	City of Glasgow		Geriatric patients and controls			
	Number in thousands	%	Number	%	Chi^2	p
Under 65	875	89	76	12		
65 and over	102	11	536	88		
Of those aged 65 and over:						
65–74	70	69	156	29	58·3	<0·01
75 and over	32	31	380	71		

Table 13 Marital status of geriatric patients, controls and population aged sixty-five and over

Marital status	City of Glasgow		Geriatric patients		Controls	
	Number in thousands	%	Number	%	Number	%
Married	42	41	143	23	209	34
Single or widowed	60	59	469	77	403	66
Total	102		612		612	

	Chi^2	p
City v. patients	20·3	<0·01
City v. controls	1·82	n.s.
Patients v. controls	17·4	<0·01

Table 14 Social characteristics of geriatric patients and of controls

Social characteristics	Geriatric patients		Controls		Chi^2	p
	Number	%	Number	%		
Lived alone	130	30	179	29		
With spouse only	80	18	131	21	1·94	n.s.
With others	229	52	302	50		
No children in locality	152	35	200	33	0·96	n.s.

134

House with bathroom	279	63	370	60	
House with WC but no bath	73	17	112	18	1·07 n.s.
House with no WC and no bath	86	20	121	20	
Other (lodging-house, etc.)	1	0·2	9	2	
Total	439		612		

Table 15   Social controls

Total number of names obtained from Executive Council	785
Of these:	
Died before research project commenced	58
Moved away; new address unknown	87
Building demolished; new address unknown	14
Moved from district; not accessible for interview	6
Age wrongly recorded	4
General practitioner unwilling to co-operate	2
Subject unwilling to co-operate	2
Number of interviews completed	612
Of these:	
Geriatric patients in survey already	13
In hospital	2
In residential home	7

Table 16   Social characteristics of geriatric patients and of medical controls

Social characteristics	Geriatric patients Number	%	Medical controls Number	%	Chi²	p
Male 65–74	26	10	73	29		
75–84	61	24	39	16		
85 and over	11	4	1	0·4		
All males	98	38	113	45	*	
Female 65–74	41	16	93	37	97·54	<0·01
75–84	79	31	36	14		
85 and over	37	15	8	3		
All females	157	62	137	55		

Married	58	23	100	40		
Single	39	15	31	12	15·6	<0·01
Widowed	158	62	119	48		
Lived alone	87	34	65	26		
With spouse only	50	20	67	27	4·36	n.s.
With others	118	46	118	47		
No children in locality	89	35	103	41	1·27	n.s.
House with bathroom	155	61	188	75		
House with WC but no bath	45	18	31	12	11·66	<0·01
House with no WC and no bath	55	21	31	12		
Social class I and II	17	7	21	8		
III	90	35	104	42	17·83	<0·01
IV and V	148	58	125	50		
Total	255		250			

*This comparison was made of the age-distribution of the two groups of patients for both sexes combined.

Table 17 Presenting symptoms of geriatric and medical patients

Medical characteristics	Geriatric patients Number	%	Medical controls Number	%	Chi²	p
Stroke	38	15	36	14	0·02	n.s.
Immobility	176	69	33	13	11·46	<0·01
Falls	120	47	39	16	162·4	<0·01
Incontinence	129	51	19	8	106·4	<0·01
Mental abnormality	125	49	13	5	112·7	<0·01
Number of symptoms:						
one	63	25	55	22		
two	67	26	18	7		
three	63	25	4	2		
four	36	14	6	2	180·7	<0·01
five	6	2	3	1		
none	20	8	164	66		
Total	255		250			

Table 18 Duration of dependency in geriatric and medical patients

Duration of dependency	Geriatric patients Number	%	Medical controls Number	%	Chi²	p
Less than one week	39	15	19	8		
One week to one month	36	14	6	2		
One month to one year	84	33	10	4	525·6	<0·01
More than one year	65	26	9	4		
Not dependent	31	12	206	82		
Total	255		250			

Table 19 Outcome—three months after admission of geriatric and medical patients

	Geriatric patients Number	%	Medical controls Number	%
Discharged	55	29	185	74
Dead	62	33	55	22
Still in hospital	72	38	10	4
Total	189		250	

Chi^2 113·2 $p < 0·01$

Table 20 Outcome three months after admission related to symptoms

Medical characteristics	Discharged				Dead				Still in hospital			
	Geriatric		Medical		Geriatric		Medical		Geriatric		Medical	
	No.	%	No.	%	No.	%	No.	%	No.	%	No.	%
Number of presenting symptoms:												
none or one	26	47	171	92	15	24	42	76	24	33	6	60
two	11	20	9	4	13	21	8	15	19	26	1	10
three, four or five	18	33	5	3	34	55	5	9	29	40	3	30
Duration of dependency:												
less than one week	11	20	9	4	5	8	6	11	9	13	4	40
one week to one month	12	22	3	2	10	16	3	5	10	14	0	0
one month to one year	12	22	8	4	19	31	2	4	27	38	0	0
more than one year	12	22	6	3	23	37	3	5	15	21	0	0
not dependent	8	15	159	86	5	7	41	75	11	15	6	60
Incontinence and mental abnormality both absent	25	45	174	94	14	23	47	85	25	35	6	60
Incontinence and mental abnormality both present	11	20	2	1	29	47	4	7	22	31	3	30
Total	55		185		62		55		72		10	

Table 21 Comparison of geriatric patients with sufficient and insufficient basic care

Social characteristics	Insufficient basic care Number	%	Sufficient care Number	%	Chi²	p
Male	33	36	80	42	0·96	n.s.
Female	58	64	109	58		
Under 65	4	4	21	11		
65–74	23	25	42	22		
75–84	46	50	95	50	3·53	n.s.
85 and over	18	19	31	16		
Married	10	11	60	32		
Single	20	22	23	12	14·54	<0·01
Widowed	61	67	106	56		
No children in locality	52	57	46	24	26·2	<0·01
Lived alone	57	62	31	16		
With spouse only	9	10	48	25	51·1	<0·01
With others	25	28	110	58		
House with bathroom	44	48	124	65		
House with WC but no bath	27	30	28	15	8·67	<0·05
House with no WC and no bath	20	22	37	20		
Social class I and II	5	5	12	6		
III	20	23	75	40	22·15	<0·01
IV and V	66	72	102	54		
Home help	46	50	30	16	37·3	<0·01
District nurse	19	21	53	28	1·71	n.s.
Meals-on-Wheels	3	3	0	0		
Total	91		189			

Table 22 Reasons for insufficient basic care

Reason	Number of subjects	%
No children in locality	52	57

Preoccupation:	health	5	
	family	2	
	employment	4	
	housing	1	
	combined	5	
		17	19

Dilemma:	children	2	
	spouse/children	1	
	personality	1	
		4	4

| Patient refused | | 7 | 7 |
| Patient rejected | | 11 | 12 |

| Total | | 91 | |

Table 23 Social characteristics of patients who received sufficient basic care with and without undue strain

Social characteristics	Undue strain Number	%	No undue strain Number	%	Chi^2	p
Male	62	44	18	38	0·60	n.s.
Female	79	56	30	62		
Under 65	19	13	2	4		
65–74	26	18	16	33	7·54	n.s.
75–84	70	50	25	52		
85 and over	26	18	5	10		
Married	47	33	13	27		
Single	13	9	10	20	5·42	n.s.
Widowed	81	58	25	52		
No children in locality	33	23	13	27	0·28	n.s.
Lived alone	18	13	13	27		
With spouse only	39	28	9	19	9·42	<0·01
With others	84	60	26	54		
House with bathroom	96	68	28	58		
House with WC but no bath	19	13	9	19	1·55	n.s.
House with no WC and no bath	26	18	11	23		

Social class I and II	11	8	1	2		
III	55	39	20	42	0·22	n.s.
IV and V	75	53	27	56		
Home help	22	16	8	17	0·13	n.s.
District nurse	44	31	9	19	2·76	n.s.
Meals-on-Wheels	0	0	0	0		
Total	141		48			

Table 24 Principal helper in cases receiving sufficient care

| | Undue strain | | No undue strain | |
	Number	%	Number	%
Principal helper				
Spouse	35	25	9	19
Own child	73	52	21	46
Child-in-law	9	6	3	6
Other family member	19	13	8	17
Neighbour	4	3	4	8
No principal helper	1	0·7	3	6
Age of principal helper				
Under 30	5	4	0	0
30–49	34	24	18	38
50–69	76	54	18	38
70 and over	25	18	9	19
No principal helper	1	0·7	3	6
Total	141		48	

Table 25 Work done by neighbours

	Number	%
Home accepted cases	280	
Helped by neighbours	47	17
Neighbour was 'principal helper'	22	8
Work done by neighbours		
Domestic only	18	38
Domestic and personal	5	11
Domestic, personal and toilet	3	6
Cleansing	21	45

Table 26 Social factors relating to help from neighbours

Social factors	Geriatric patients	Help from neighbours Number	%
Male	113	11	10
Female	167	36	22
Aged under 75	90	14	16
75 and over	190	33	17
Social class I and II	17	3	18
III	95	12	13
IV and V	168	32	39
Housing: pensioners'	18	5	28
other Corporation	110	10	9
private with bath	40	7	18
WC but no bath	48	4	8
no WC and no bath	57	18	32
hostel	7	3	42
Total	280	47	17

Table 27 Use of domiciliary services by geriatric patients

	Subjects using services Number	%
Home help	76	27
District nurse	72	25
Meals-on-Wheels	3	1
Number of subjects	280	

Table 28 Social characteristics and use of domiciliary services

Social characteristics	Geriatric patients	Attended by home help Number	%	Attended by district nurse Number	%
Male	113	17	15	27	24
Female	167	59	35	45	27
Under 65	25	3	12	9	36
65–74	65	13	20	8	12
75–84	141	39	28	42	30
85 and over	49	21	43	13	27

Married	70	14	20	22	31
Single	43	16	37	8	19
Widowed	167	46	28	42	25
Lived alone	88	45	51	18	20
With spouse only	57	14	25	21	37
With others	135	17	13	33	24
No children in locality	98	45	45	24	24
Total	280	76		72	

Table 29 Medical characteristics and use of domiciliary services

Medical characteristics	Geriatric patients	Attended by home help		Attended by district nurse	
		Number	%	Number	%
Stroke	43	5	12	15	35
Immobility	195	58	30	62	31
Falls	130	41	32	31	24
Incontinence	108	24	22	34	31
Mental abnormality	134	25	19	35	26
Number of symptoms:					
one	73	23	32	14	19
two	73	21	29	19	26
three	68	22	32	19	28
four	38	4	11	12	32
five	7	1	14	4	57
none	21	5	25	4	20
Duration of dependency:					
less than one week	43	14	33	11	26
one week to one month	37	9	24	7	19
one month to one year	90	25	27	26	29
more than one year	77	17	23	22	28
not dependent	33	11	33	6	18
Total	280	76		72	

Table 30 Use of domiciliary services by geriatric patients related to basic care and strain

	Geriatric patients	Attended by home help		Attended by district nurse	
		Number	%	Number	%
Sufficient basic care	189	30	16	53	28
Insufficient basic care	91	46	50	19	21
No undue strain	48	8	17	9	19
Undue strain	141	22	16	44	30

Table 31 Insufficient basic care

Lack of	Number of subjects
Food only	0
Warmth only	0
Cleanliness only	5
Safety only	22
Food and warmth	1
Food and cleanliness	0
Food and safety	2
Warmth and cleanliness	4
Warmth and safety	2
Cleanliness and safety	11
Food, warmth and cleanliness	6
Food, warmth and safety	2
Food, cleanliness and safety	8
Warmth, cleanliness and safety	1
Food, warmth, cleanliness and safety	27
Total	91

Table 32 Comparison of presenting symptoms in patients with sufficient and insufficient basic care

Medical characteristics	Insufficient basic care Number	%	Sufficient care Number	%	Chi²	p
Stroke	5	5	38	20	10·1	<0·01
Falls	49	54	81	43	2·99	n.s.
Immobility	56	62	139	74	4·18	<0·05
Incontinence	35	38	73	39	0·01	n.s.
Mental abnormality	35	38	99	52	4·76	<0·05
Number of symptoms:						
one	21	23	52	28		
two	29	32	44	23		
three	26	29	42	22	11·75	<0·05
four	5	5	33	17		
five	1	1	6	3		
none	9	10	12	6		
Duration of dependency:						
less than one week	12	13	31	16		
one week to one month	12	13	25	13		
one month to one year	34	37	56	30	2·76	n.s.
more than one year	21	23	56	30		
not dependent	12	13	21	11		
Total	91		189			

Table 33 Comparison of presenting symptoms in patients who received sufficient basic care with and without undue strain

Medical characteristics	Undue strain Number	%	No undue strain Number	%	Chi²	p
Stroke	26	18	12	25	0·95	n.s.
Falls	62	44	19	40	0·28	n.s.
Immobility	106	75	33	69	0·76	n.s.
Incontinence	61	43	12	25	5·03	<0·05
Mental abnormality	79	56	20	42	2·96	n.s.

Number of symptoms:

one	39	28	13	27		
two	33	23	11	23		
three	30	21	12	25	5·75	n.s.
four	28	20	5	10		
five	5	4	1	2		
none	6	4	6	13		

Duration of dependency:

less than one week	20	14	11	20		
one week to one month	16	11	9	19		
one month to one year	47	33	9	19	12·82	<0·05
more than one year	47	33	9	19		
not dependent	11	8	10	20		
Total	141		48			

Table 34 Work done by home helps

	Number	%
Domestic only	24	32
Domestic and personal	10	13
Domestic, personal and toilet	12	16
Cleansing	30	39
Total	76	

Table 35 Survey of incontinence

Of the last 100 consecutive cases in the main survey, twenty had been frequently incontinent of urine for two or more days.

The following information was obtained from this sample:
 8 had been incontinent for more than three months.
 5 were incontinent of faeces.

9   did *not* have incontinence pads.
4   disposed of pads in dustbin.
8   were *not* visited by the district nurse.
1   sent linen to a commercial laundry.
2   used a commercial laundrette.
1   was aware of the Local Authority laundry service.
0   received financial assistance with laundry from the Ministry of Social Security.
6   washed linen away from patient's house.
10 washed linen at patient's house with adequate facilities.
4   washed linen at patient's house with inadequate facilities (no hot water).

Persons performing washing or laundry procedures:

for nine female patients		*for eleven male patients*	
self	1	spouse	5
home help	2	daughter	3
daughter	4	niece	2
nephew	1	daughter-in-law	1
daughter-in-law	1		

Table 36   Survey of final illness

Place of death	Number of subjects	% of all deaths
At home	2,731	35·2
On holiday	13	0·2
Residential home	297	3·9
Public place	28	0·4
Dead on arrival at hospital	149	2·0
Nursing home	179	2·3
Hospital: medical	1,929	25·4
surgical	853	11·2
geriatric	1,101	14·5
psychiatric	327	4·3
All hospitals	4,210	55·4
All deaths	7,607	

Table 37 Place of death by age and sex

	Home Number	%	Hospital Number	%	Elsewhere Number	%	All deaths
Males 65–74	678	36·1	1,080	57·6	118	6·3	1,876
75–84	399	32·9	703	58·0	111	9·2	1,213
85 and over	126	34·8	185	51·1	51	14·1	362
All males	1,203	34·9	1,968	57·0	280	8·1	3,451
Females 65–74	561	36·0	903	58·0	93	6·0	1,557
75–84	645	35·9	976	54·3	176	9·6	1,797
85 and over	322	40·1	363	45·3	117	14·6	802
All females	1,528	36·7	2,242	53·9	386	8·3	4,156
Both sexes 65–74	1,239	36·1	1,983	57·8	211	6·1	3,433
75–84	1,044	34·7	1,679	55·8	287	9·5	3,010
85 and over	448	38·5	548	47·1	168	14·4	1,164
Total	2,731	35·2	4,210	55·3	666	8·8	7,607

Table 38 Type of ward in which death occurred related to age and sex

Social characteristics		Medical	Surgical	Geriatric	Psychiatric	Total
Males	65–74	644	215	160	61	1,080
	75–84	276	150	218	59	703
	85 and over	46	27	94	18	185
All males		966	392	462	138	1,968
Females	65–74	491	224	141	47	903
	75–84	393	177	323	83	976
	85 and over	79	60	165	59	363
All females		963	461	629	189	2,242
Both sexes	65–74	1,135	439	301	108	1,983
	75–84	669	327	541	142	1,679
	85 and over	125	87	259	77	548
Total		1,929	853	1,101	327	4,210

Summary

Age group (both sexes)	% of deaths	
	Medical and surgical	Geriatric and psychiatric
65–74	46	12
75–84	33	23
85 and over	18	29

149

Table 39 Place of death by marital status

Social characteristics		Home Number	%	Hospital Number	%	Elsewhere Number	%	All deaths
Males	Married	702	38·6	1,027	56·5	90	4·9	1,819
	Single	102	24·8	253	61·4	57	13·8	412
	Widowed	399	32·7	688	56·4	133	10·9	1,220
All males		1,203	34·9	1,968	57·0	280	8·1	3,451
Females	Married	290	39·6	409	55·8	34	4·6	733
	Single	237	30·1	427	54·3	123	15·6	787
	Widowed	1,001	38·0	1,406	53·3	229	8·7	2,636
All females		1,528	36·7	2,242	53·9	386	9·3	4,156
Both sexes	Married	992	38·9	1,436	56·3	124	4·9	2,552
	Single	339	28·3	680	56·7	180	15·0	1,199
	Widowed	1,400	36·3	2,094	54·2	362	9·4	3,856
Total		2,731	35·2	4,210	55·3	666	8·8	7,607

Table 40 Type of ward in which death occurred related to marital status

Marital Status	Medical and surgical		Geriatric and psychiatric		All deaths
	Number	%	Number	%	
Married	1,080	42·3	356	13·9	2,552
Single	407	33·9	273	22·8	1,199
Widowed	1,295	33·6	799	20·7	3,856
All deaths	2,782	36·6	1,428	18·8	7,607

Table 41 Social class and place of death

Social class	Home		Hospital		Elsewhere		All deaths
	Number	%	Number	%	Number	%	
I	80	39·6	89	44·1	33	16·3	202
II	330	35·3	492	52·6	114	12·2	936
III	1,223	39·3	1,659	53·3	232	7·5	3,114
IV	658	30·8	1,319	61·8	157	7·4	2,134
V	365	39·2	483	51·9	82	8·8	930
Not classified	75	25·8	168	57·7	48	16·5	291
All deaths	2,731	35·2	4,210	55·3	666	8·8	7,607

Table 42 Type of ward in which death occurred related to social class

Social class	Medical and surgical Number	%	Geriatric and psychiatric Number	%	All deaths
I	62	30·7	27	13·4	202
II	338	36·1	154	16·5	936
III	1,112	35·7	547	17·6	3,114
IV	867	40·6	452	21·2	2,134
V	325	35·3	158	17·2	920
Not classified	78	26·8	90	30·9	291
All deaths	2,782	36·6	1,428	18·8	7,607

Table 43 Duration of hospital stay related to age and sex

Age and sex		Number of hospital deaths	Total hospital bed-days	Average duration of stay (days)	% of total hospital bed-days
Males	65–74	1,080	91,200	84	14
	75–84	703	126,936	181	19
	85 and over	185	40,236	212	6
Females	65–74	903	76,571	85	12
	75–84	976	178,193	183	27
	85 and over	363	144,933	399	22
All deaths		4,210	658,069	156	100

Table 44 Duration of hospital stay related to type of ward

Type of ward	Number of deaths	Total hospital bed-days	Average duration of stay (days)	% of deaths	% of bed-days
Medical	1,929	59,019	31	46	9
Surgical	853	23,484	28	20	4
Geriatric	1,101	229,251	208	26	35
Psychiatric	327	345,245	1,056	8	52
All hospitals	4,210	656,999	156	100	100

Table 45 Hospital bed-days per death

Age and sex		Number of deaths	Total hospital bed-days	Hospital bed-days per death	Hospital beds occupied
Males	65–74	1,876	91,200	49	249
	75–84	1,213	126,936	105	347
	85 and over	362	40,236	111	110
Females	65–74	1,557	76,571	49	209
	75–84	1,797	178,193	99	487
	85 and over	802	144,933	181	396
All deaths		7,607	658,069	86	1,798

Table 46 Deaths in nursing homes

Social characteristics		Deaths in nursing homes	% of all deaths in each group
All deaths		179	2·4
All males		47	1·4
All females		132	3·2
Both sexes:	65–74	49	1·4
	75–84	87	2·8
	85 and over	43	3·7
Married		25	1·0
Single		52	4·3
Widowed		102	2·6
Social class:			
I		20	9·9
II		53	5·7
III		47	1·5
IV		26	1·2
V		18	1·9
0 (no occupation or not known)		15	5·1

Table 47 Deaths in residential homes

Social characteristics		Deaths in homes	% of all deaths in each group
All deaths		297	3·9
Males		121	3·5
Females		176	4·2
Both sexes	65–74	49	1·4
	75–84	136	4·4
	85 and over	112	9·6
Married		18	0·7
Single		96	8·0
Widowed		183	4·8
Social class:			
I		11	5·4
II		45	4·8
III		115	3·7
IV		65	3·0
V		38	4·1
0 (no occupation or not known)		23	7·9

Table 48 Dead on arrival at hospital

Age and sex		Dead on arrival	% of all deaths
All deaths		149	2·0
Males		88	2·6
Females		61	1·5
Both sexes	65–74	89	2·6
	75–84	50	1·7
	85 and over	10	0·9

Table 49 Comparison between samples in final illness survey

Social characteristics		% of subjects in sample Sub-sample (240)	Main sample (7,607)
Male		48	45
Female		52	55
Both sexes	65–74	51	45
	75–84	36	40
	85 and over	14	15
Married		39	34
Single		12	16
Widowed		49	50
Died at home		44	35
Died in hospital		56	55
Died elsewhere		excluded	10
Type of ward in which death occurred:			
medical		28	25
surgical		11	11
geriatric		14	15
psychiatric		3	4

Table 50 Survey of final illness

			Number of subjects
Interview obtained with:	spouse	44	
	other relative	145	
	neighbour	25	214
No contact with relatives or neighbours, but information obtained from:			
	hospital records	23	
	general practitioner	2	
	minister of religion	1	
			26
Refused interview			10
Total			250
Interval between death and interview:			
	less than 2 months		15
	2–3 months		3
	3–4 months		30

4–5 months	55
5–6 months	55
6–7 months	56
Total	214

Number of calls before contact was made (including ten who refused):

one	144
two	60
three or four	14
five or more	6
Total	224

Table 51 Comparison of subjects who died at home and in hospital

Social characteristics	Subjects who died			
	At home		In hospital	
	Number	%	Number	%
Male	47	44	69	51
Female	59	56	65	49
Age 65–74	59	56	62	46
75–84	36	34	50	37
85 and over	11	10	22	16
Married	41	39	52	39
Single	11	10	19	14
Widowed	54	51	63	47
No children in locality	28	26	51	38
Lived alone	24	22	34	25
With spouse only	24	22	33	25
With others	58	55	67	50
Number of subjects	106		134	

Table 52 Symptoms and duration of dependency related to place of death

Symptoms and duration	Home		Hospital	
	Number	%	Number	%
Immobility	69	65	76	59
Incontinence	42	40	45	34
Mental abnormality	18	17	52	39

Duration of dependency:

not dependent	34	32	40	28
less than one week	22	21	15	12
one week to one month	12	11	17	13
one month to one year	22	20	30	23
more than one year	16	16	32	24
Number of subjects	106		134	

Table 53 Symptoms and duration of dependency related to age

Symptoms and duration	% of subjects			
	65–74	75–84	85 and over	All ages
Immobility	56	63	70	60
Incontinence	35	34	48	36
Mental abnormality	18	34	51	29
Duration of dependency:				
not dependent	39	26	15	31
less than one month	25	31	27	27
one month to one year	21	21	27	22
more than one year	16	22	31	20

TABLE 54 Survey of final illness and principal helper

	Subjects who died		
	At home	In hospital	Total
Spouse	28	32	60
Son or daughter	38	31	69
Other family member	10	22	32
Neighbour or friend	10	15	25
No principal helper	20	34	54
Age of principal helper:			
under 30	1	4	5
30–49	37	24	61
50–69	35	43	78
70 and over	13	29	42

Table 55 Domiciliary services

| | Subjects who died | | | | | |
| | At home | | In hospital | | Total | |
	Number	%	Number	%	Number	%
Home help	8	8	19	14	27	11
District nurse	20	19	12	9	32	13
Meals-on-Wheels	0	0	1	0·7	1	0·4
Number of subjects	106		134		240	
(Six subjects had more than one service.)						
For subjects who were dependent for more than one month:						
Home help	5	13	16	26	21	21
District nurse	11	29	8	13	19	19
Meals-on-Wheels	0	0	1	2	1	1
Number of subjects	38		62		100	
(Six subjects had more than one service.)						

Table 56   Use of domiciliary services related to age of subject

Age	Number of subjects	% who used	
		Home helps	District nurse
65–74	121	7	14
75–84	86	15	16
85 and over	33	18	3
All ages	240	11	13

Table 57 Projected need of hospital beds for final hospitalization and of domiciliary services for final illness of population of Scotland aged sixty-five and over

	Age group			Total population aged 65 and over
	65–74	75–84	85 and over	
Total deaths in each age group in 1968 (a)	17,334	17,429	7,845	42,608
Average bed-days per death in 1968 (b)	49	102	146	—
Beds utilized: $\frac{a \times b}{*366}$ (c)	2,321	4,857	3,129	—
Population in 1968	402,400	174,000	32,600	609,000
Projected population in 1981	443,000	215,000	37,000	695,000
Percentage increase (d)	10	24	13	—
Additional beds required (d of c)	232	1,166	407	1,805
Increase in number of deaths (d of a)	1,733	4,183	1,020	6,936
Percentage who utilized home helps	7	15	18	—
Increase in number of subjects utilizing home helps	121	627	184	932
Percentage who utilized district nurses	14	16	3	—
Increase in number of subjects utilizing district nurses	242	669	31	942

*Leap year

Bibliography

The following publications are scientific accounts of material presented in this volume:

Isaacs, B. (1966). 'Measuring the demand for geriatric beds', *Medical Care*, vol. 4, no. 4.

—— (1969a). 'Some characteristics of geriatric patients', *Scottish Med. J.*, vol. 14, p. 243.

—— (1969b). 'Housing for old people: the view of a geriatrician', *Journal of the Institute of Housing Managers*, vol. 5, no. 4.

—— (1970). 'Changes in the demand for geriatric care', *Geront. clin.*, vol. 12, p. 257.

—— (1971a). *Studies of Illness and Death in the Elderly in Glasgow.* (a) *Survival of the Unfittest.* (b) *Life Before Death.* Scottish Health Service Study no. 17.

—— (1971b). 'Geriatric patients: do their families care?', *Brit. Med. J.*, 4, pp. 282-6.

—— (1972). 'Towards a definition of geriatrics', *J. chron. Dis.*, (in the press).

Isaacs, B. *et al.* (1971). 'The concept of pre-death', *Lancet*, i, p. 1115.

The following books and articles, mostly from British and American literature, are among many works in geriatric medicine and social gerontology which have exerted an influence on the formation of the authors' ideas:

Geriatric medicine

Anderson, W. F. & Isaacs, B. (eds) (1964). *Current Achievements in Geriatrics.* London, Cassell.

Blessed, G., Tomlinson, B. E. & Roth, M. (1968). 'The association between quantitative measures of dementia and of senile change in the cerebral grey matter of elderly subjects', *Brit. J. Psychiat.*, vol. 114, pp. 797–812.

Burvill, P. W. (1970). 'Physical illness in the elderly: a study of patients in mental hospitals, geriatric hospitals and nursing homes', *Geront. clin.*, vol. 12, p. 288.

Gray, B. (1966). *Home Accidents among Old People: Report of a Research*

Carried out in the Birmingham Area. Royal Society for the Prevention of Accidents.

Hughes, W. (1970). 'Alzheimer's disease', *Geront. clin.*, vol. 12, pp. 129–48.

Macmillan, D. & Shaw, P. (1966). 'Senile breakdown in standards of personal and environmental cleanliness', *Brit. Med. J.*, ii, p. 1032.

Roth, M. (1955). 'The natural history of mental disorders in old age', *J. ment. Sci.*, vol. 101, pp. 281-301.

Sheldon, J. H. (1960). 'On the natural history of falls in old age', *Brit. Med. J.*, ii, pp. 1685–90.

Snellgrove, D. R. (1963). *Elderly Housebound: A Report on Elderly People who are Incapacitated.* Luton, White Crescent Press.

Wilson, L. A., Lawson, I. R. & Brass, W. (1962). 'Multiple disorders in the elderly', *Lancet*, ii, p. 841.

Medical care

Anderson, W. F. & Cowan, N. R. (1955). 'A consultative health centre for older people', *Lancet*, ii, p. 239.

Arnold, J. & Exton-Smith, A. N. (1962). 'The geriatric department and the community: value of hospital treatment in the elderly', *Lancet*, ii, p. 551.

Binks, F. A. (1968). 'Approach to disability and breakdown', *Brit. Med. J.*, i, pp. 269-74.

Brocklehurst, J. C. (1964). 'The work of a geriatric day hospital', *Geront. clin.*, vol. 6, p. 151.

Brocklehurst, J. C. & Shergold, M. (1968). 'What happens when geriatric patients leave hospital?', *Lancet*, ii, pp. 1133–5.

—— (1969). 'Old people leaving hospital', *Geront. clin.*, vol. 11, p. 115.

Burns, C. (1969). 'Geriatric care in general practice: a medico-social survey of 391 patients undertaken by Health Visitors', *J. Royal Coll. General Practitioners*, vol. 18, p. 287.

Droller, H. (1969). 'Does community care really reach the elderly sick?', *Geront. clin.*, vol. 11, p. 169.

Ferguson, T. & Macphail, A. N. (1954). *Hospital and Community*, published for the Nuffield Provincial Hospitals Trust by Oxford University Press.

Glyn Hughes, H. L. (1960). *Peace at the last: A Survey of Terminal Care in the United Kingdom.* A report to the Gulbenkian Foundation, London.

HMSO (1966). Scottish Hospitals Survey. *Report in the Western Region.* Department of Health for Scotland, Edinburgh.

HMSO (1970). *Services for the Elderly with Mental Disorder.* Report of a sub-committee at the Standing Medical Advisory Committee of the Scottish Health Services Council.

Hobson, W. & Pemberton, J. (1955). *The Health of the Elderly at Home: A Medical, Social and Dietary Study of Elderly People Living at Home in Sheffield.* London, Butterworth.

Hoenig, J. & Hamilton, M. W. (1967). 'The burden on the household in an extra-mural psychiatric service', in H. Freeman & J. Farndale (eds), *New Aspects of the Mental Health Services* (Westminster Series, vol. 7), Pergamon Press, pp. 612–35.

Kay, D. W. K., Beamish, P. & Roth, M. (1962). 'Some medical and social characteristics of elderly people under state care: a comparison of geriatric wards, mental hospitals and welfare homes', in *Sociology and Medicine: Studies within the Framework of the British National Health Service*, Sociological Review, monograph 5. University of Keele.

—— (1964). 'Old age mental disorders in Newcastle-upon-Tyne', *Brit. J. Psychiat.*, vol. 110, p. 146.

Kay, D. W. K., Roth, M. & Hall, M. R. P. (1966). 'Special problems of the aged and the organization of hospital services', *Brit. Med. J.*, ii, p. 967.

Lowenthal, M. (1966). *Lives in Distress: The Paths of the Elderly to the Psychiatric Ward*. New York, Basic Books.

Lowther, C. P., MacLeod, R. D. M. & Williamson, J. (1970). 'Evaluation of early diagnostic services for the elderly', *Brit. Med. J.*, 3, pp. 275–7.

Lowther, C. P. & Williamson, J. (1966). 'Old people and their relatives', *Lancet*, ii, pp. 1459–60.

Mackay, J. S. B. & Ruck, S. K. (1967). *The Care of the Aged in the Manchester Regional Hospital Board Area*. Manchester Regional Hospital Board.

McNabola, E. K. A. (1970). *An Assessment of the Elderly by a District Nursing Sister Attached to a Group Practice*. Scottish Health Bulletin, vol. 28, no. 9.

Martin, F. M. (1962). *Trends in Psycho-geriatric Care*. London, PEP Broadsheets, vol. 32, no. 497, pp. 163–94.

Mezey, A. G., Hodkinson, H. A. & Evans, G. J. (1968). 'The elderly in the wrong unit', *Brit. Med. J.*, 3, pp. 16–19.

Miller, H. C. (1963). *The Ageing Countryman: A Social and Medical Report on Old Age in a Country Practice*. National Corporation for the Care of Old People.

Morton, E. V. B., Barker, M. E. & MacMillan, D. (1968). 'The joint assessment and early treatment unit in psycho-geriatric care', *Geront. clin.*, vol. 10, pp. 65–73.

Nisbet, N. H. (1962). 'A review of 1,000 elderly patients awaiting admission to hospital', *Lancet*, ii, pp. 770–3.

—— (1967). 'How long is long-term?', *Scot. Med. J.*, vol. 12, p. 223.

—— (1970). 'Who benefits?', *Lancet*, i, p. 133.

Nisbet, N. H., Mackenzie, M. S. & Hamilton, M. C. (1966). 'Follow-up of elderly discharged patients', *Lancet*, i, p. 1314.

Norton, D. (1967). *Hospitals and the Long-stay Patient*. London, Pergamon Press.

Parnell, R. W. (1968). 'Prospective geriatric bed requirements in a mental hospital', *Geront. clin.*, vol. 10, pp. 30–6.

Sheldon, J. H. (1948). *Social Medicine in Old Age*. London, Oxford University Press.

Silver, C. P. & Zuberi, S. J. (1965). 'Prognosis of patients admitted to a geriatric unit', *Geront. clin.*, vol. 7, p. 348.

Silberstein, J. *et al.* (1970). 'Causes of admission to nursing homes in Israel', *Medical Care*, vol. VIII, p. 3.

Stewart, M. (1968). *My Brother's Keeper?* London, Health Horizon.

Thomas, P. (1968). 'Experiences of two preventive clinics for the elderly', *Brit. Med. J.*, 2, pp. 357–60.

Warren, M. D. (1964). 'Demands and needs for inpatient care for elderly people', *Medical Care*, vol. 2, p. 113.

Williamson, J. (1963). *The Care of the Elderly in Scotland*. Edinburgh, Royal College of Physicians.

—— (1970). *The Care of the Elderly in Scotland: a follow-up report*. Edinburgh, Royal College of Physicians.

Williamson, J. *et al.* (1964). 'Old people at home: their unreported needs', *Lancet*, i, p. 1117.

World Health Organization (1959). Technical Report Series 171.

Social gerontology

Brockington, F. & Lempert, S. (1966). *The Social Needs of the Over-80's*. Manchester University Press.

Cumming, E. & Henry, W. E. (1961). *Growing Old: The Process of Disengagement*. New York, Basic Books.

Cunnison, J. *et al.* (1958). *The Third Statistical Account of Scotland: Glasgow*. Glasgow, Collins.

Exton-Smith, A. N. & Stanton, B. A. (1965). *Report of an Investigation into the Dietary of Elderly Women Living Alone*. London, King Edward's Hospital Fund.

Farndale, J. (ed.) (1965). *Trends in Social Welfare*. London, Pergamon Press.

Morris, J. N. *et al.* (1966). 'Our old people: next steps in social policy', *Socialist Commentary*.

Richardson, I. M. (1964). *Age and Need: A Study of Older People in North-East Scotland*. Edinburgh, Livingstone.

Rose, A. M. & Peterson, W. A. (eds.) (1965). *Older People and their Social World: The Sub-culture of the Aging*. Philadelphia, F. A. Davis.

Shanas, E. *et al.* (1968). *Old People in Three Industrial Societies*. London, Routledge & Kegan Paul.

Townsend, P. (1957). *The Family Life of Old People*. London, Routledge & Kegan Paul.

Townsend, P. & Wedderburn, D. (1965). *The Aged in the Welfare State*. London, Bell.

Tunstall, J. (1966). *Old and Alone: A Sociological Study of Old People*. London, Routledge & Kegan Paul.

Twaddle, A. C. (1968). 'Aging, population growth and chronic illness: a projection, United States, 1960–1985', *J. chron. Dis.*, vol. 21, pp. 417–22.

Williams, Lady Gertrude (1969). *The New Challenge in Social Welfare*. Glasgow, Berl Wober Memorial Lecture.

Williams, R. H., Tibbits, C. and Donahue, W. (1963). *Processes of Aging: Social and Psychological Perspective*, vol. 2, p. 272. New York, Atherton Press.

Young, M. & Willmott, P. (1957). *Family and Kinship in East London*. London, Routledge & Kegan Paul.

165

Social care

Carstairs, V. (1966). *Home Nursing in Scotland: Report of an Inquiry into the Local Authority Domiciliary Services.* Scottish Health Service Studies, vol. 2, Scottish Home and Health Dept.

Harris, A. I. (1968). *Social Welfare for the Elderly.* London, HMSO.

Sumner, G. & Smith, R. (1970). *Planning Local Authority Services for the Elderly.* London, Allen & Unwin.

Townsend, P. (1962). *The Last Refuge: A Survey of Residential Institutions and Homes for the Aged in England and Wales.* London, Routledge & Kegan Paul.

Wedderburn, D. (1966). 'A new look at the services needed', *Quarterly Bulletin* of the National Old People's Welfare Council.

Williams, G. (1967). *Caring for People: Staffing Residential Homes. Report of the Committee of Enquiry set up by the National Council of Social Service.* London, Allen & Unwin.

Index

Adaptation of homes, 13
Admission
  to geriatric unit, 14
  intermittent, 102
  of old people to hospital, 2, 9, 12, 14, 23-7
Age distribution of medical and geriatric patients, 17
Alcohol, 5, 31, 45-7
Alstead, Professor Stanley, 11
Amulree, Lord, 11
Anderson, Professor W. Ferguson, 11, 12, 22, 99
Atherosclerosis, 75, 95
Atmospheric pollution, 7, 95

'Bar', 9, 10
Barnhill, 10, 11
'Basic care', 23, 109
Birmingham, population density, 6
Blindness, 40, 42
Brocklehurst, Professor John, 11
Brown, O. T., 11
Burns, C., 99

Camden, London Borough of, 102
Cerebral arteriosclerosis, 56
Chiropody, 13, 14, 88
Churches, 6, 101
Cleanliness, lack of, 29, 31
Clubs for retired people, 101
Colostomy, 40
Community, 20, 25, 71, 84-92
Confusion, 18, 19, 29

Conjugal life, disturbance of, as cause of strain, 68
Control group, 16, 107
Convalescent holidays, 14
Corporation of Glasgow
  domiciliary and residential services, 104
  Home Help services, 84
  hospitals, 8
  housing estates, 5
Cowan, Nairn, 22, 99

Day Centre, 88
Day hospital, 13, 88, 99, 102
Deafness, 98
Deaths
  before admission, 14
  in geriatric unit, 14, 18
  in medical unit, 18
  survey, 71-5
Dementia, 18, 19, 31, 75, 95
Dependency, 3, 18, 73, 98
Depression, 61, 98
Diagnosis, 12
'Dilemma', 35, 40-4
Disability in final illness, 74
Discharges
  geriatric unit, 14, 18
  medical unit, 18
Disorientation, 59
District nurses, 14, 33, 53, 69, 74, 82, 87-9, 99
Domiciliary assessment visit, 14
Domiciliary services, 8, 88
  projected future needs, 94, 113

Duration
   of dependency, 18 (before
      death), 73
   of stay (in geriatric wards), 15
      (in hospital before death), 72

Early diagnosis clinics, 22
East End of Glasgow, 4-7
   population, 6
Education, 95
   of district nurses, 100, 102
   of medical students, 100
   post graduate, 100
Electricity, danger, 29, 31
Emigration, 1, 6
Employment
   as a cause of insufficient care, 38
   as a cause of strain, 66-7
England and Wales, population, 6
Eventide Home, 3

Falls, 1, 18, 28, 30, 52, 56, 63, 105
Family doctor service, 8
Fire danger, 29, 31
Flatlets, warden-service, 6
Food, lack, 29, 31
Foresthall, 11, 12
Fracture of neck of femur, 19, 100

Galbraith, J. K., 22
Gas, danger, 29, 31
General practitioner, 8, 17, 88, 98-9
Geriatrics, 11, 16, 22
Geriatric medicine, Glasgow Royal
      Infirmary Department of, 2,
      13-15, 104
Geriatric patients, survey, 2, 16
Geriatric sub-committee of Western
      Regional Hospital Board, 12
Geriatric units, 11, 12
   deaths in, 72
Glasgow
   District Nursing Association, 87
   geography, 4-6
   geriatric services, 12
   Health and Welfare Department,
      13, 110
   housing, 4-6
   Old People's Welfare Committee,
      13
   population, 6, 104
   Retirement Council, 99

Glasgow Royal Infirmary, 8, 14
'Good Neighbour' service, 89, 101,
      102

'Hard core', 20-2
Health centres, 99, 102
Health visitors, 14, 82, 99, 100
Health and Welfare Department,
      Corporation of Glasgow, 13,
      110
Heart disease, 36
Help from relatives, 53, 63-70
Holiday admissions, 14
Home, deaths at, 73
Home help, 2, 13, 28, 30, 32, 33,
      36, 53, 69, 74, 82, 84-8, 100
Hospitals, 8-11
Hospital Admissions Department, 9
Hospital beds available, 104
'Hospital bed-days per death', 72
Hospital services, projected future
      needs, 93, 113
Houses, pensioners, 6
Housing
   as a cause of insufficient care, 38
   as a cause of strain, 67
   estate, 5
   Glasgow, 4-6
   of geriatric patients, 17, 90-1
   of old people, 91, 97
   sheltered, 6, 91, 96
   three-generation, 68
Hypothermia, 32

Inability to walk, 18, 52, 73, 105
'Inadequate personality', 64
Incontinence, 18, 29, 31, 41, 51, 56,
      60, 73, 78, 80-3, 95, 105, 109
   estimated prevalence, 80
   pads, 30, 51, 81
   survey, 80, 109
Insufficient basic care, 25, 28-33,
Isolation, 32   [109

Laundry services, 82, 88, 102
'Life space', 65-7
Living alone, 17, 34
Local Authority services, 8, 13, 82,
      99
London, population density, 6
Long-stay geriatric units, 3, 12, 13,
      15, 33
Luncheon clubs, 13, 88

McNabola, E. K. A., 99
Malnutrition, 32, 98
Marital status of medical and geriatric patients, 17
Marriage, second, 47, 64
Meals on Wheels, 13, 14, 32, 88, 101
Medical characteristics
  geriatric patients, 24, 33, 53
  medical and geriatric patients, 16, 108
  persons dying at home and in hospital, 74
Medical need, 26
Medical social work, 13
Medical unit
  deaths in, 72
  patients admitted, 16, 108
'Medical urgency', 25
Memory, loss of, 59
Mental abnormality, 18-20, 52, 59, 73, 105
  as cause of strain, 57-61
Morris, Professor Noah, 11
Mortality of medical and geriatric patients, 18
Multiple sclerosis, 57, 68
Multi-storey housing blocks, 4, 6

Neglect, 34, 45
Neighbours, 1-3, 65, 89-90
'Night sitters', 88
Nisbet, Nanette, 11
Nursing homes, 110
Nursing services, 102

Occupancy of geriatric beds, 15
Occupational therapy, domiciliary, 13, 14, 88
Old people's homes, 13
Old People's Welfare Committee, 13
Osteoarthritis, 66
Outcome of hospital treatment, 18, 106
Outpatient services, 13, 14, 99

Parkinson's disease, 29, 86
Pensioners' houses, 6
Personality of patient, as cause of strain, 61
Physical incapacity, as cause of strain, 55
Physiotherapy, domiciliary, 13, 88

Place of death of old people, 71-5, 76
Planning, 95
Pollution, atmospheric, 7, 95
Poor Law Institution, 10
Population
  density, 6
  Glasgow, 6
  projections, Scotland, 73, 93
  sample, characteristics, 16
Poverty, 7
'Preoccupation', 35-9
Pre-retirement training, 94, 99
Preventive services, 8
'Principal helpers', 63-5
Prostitution, 46, 47
Psychiatric disturbances in relatives, 64
Psychiatric services, 10, 19, 100
Psychiatric unit
  deaths in, 72
  referrals to, 14, 107
Psycho-geriatric assessment units, 100
Public Health Department, 9

Recluses, 31
Red Cross, 13
Refresher courses for district nurses, 100
'Refusal', 35, 42-4
Regional Hospital Board, 8
Rehabilitation, 15, 100
'Rejection', 35, 45-9
Relatives, help from, 70
'Relief of strain', 25
Research, 95, 96, 102
Residential homes, 13, 14, 91, 107
Rheumatoid arthritis, 39, 55, 57, 75
Rota of patient care, 69
Royal College of Physicians of Edinburgh, Report, 98
Rutherglen clinic, 22, 99

Safety, lack of, 29, 30, 31
Scotland
  population, 6
  social services, 104
Screening, 22
Sickness benefit, 66
Single state, 17
Sleep, loss of, as a cause of strain, 56

Slums in Glasgow, 4
Social characteristics
  geriatric patients, 24, 33, 53
  medical and geriatric patients, 16, 109
  persons dying at home and in hospital, 72
Social class, geriatric patients, 17
Social consequences of illness, 24
Social need, 26
Social services, 13, 109
Social Work (Scotland) Act, 13
Social workers, 13, 101, 105
Southern General Hospital, Glasgow, 11
Speech therapy, 14
Stobhill Hospital, Glasgow, 9, 11
Strain on relatives, 50-70, 109
Stroke, 18, 24, 36, 37, 100, 105
Sub-nutrition, 7
Surgical units, deaths in, 72
Survey
  final illness, 71, 109
  geriatric patients, 2, 104-13
  incontinent patients, 78, 109
Survival of patients in geriatric unit, 15
Survival of the unfittest, 3, 77

Tenements, 4
'Therapeutic optimism', 23
Toilets
  inside, 5
  outside, 2, 4, 29

Transfer of patients from general wards to geriatric unit, 14, 15, 18
'Triangles of dependency', 76

Under-occupation of houses, 5
Universities
  chairs in geriatric medicine, 95
  research, 102
University of Glasgow, Department of Materia Medica and Therapeutics, 9
Unmet need, 27

Visiting services, 13, 14
Voluntary hospitals, 8
Voluntary organizations, 6, 13, 100, 101, 104

Waiting time for admission to geriatric unit, 14
Wandering, 19, 29
Warden-service flatlets, 6, 96
Warmth, lack of, 29
Warren, Marjorie, 11
Western Regional Hospital Board, 11, 12, 13
Widowed state, 17, 64
Williamson, J., 22, 99
Women's Royal Voluntary Services, 13

'Young chronic sick', 19, 107